PSYCHOTIC DISORDERS
A Practical Guide

OTHER PRACTICAL GUIDES IN PSYCHIATRY

- **Alzheimer Disease and Other Dementias**
- **Child and Adolescent Psychiatry**
- **Mood Disorders**
- **Psychosomatic Medicine**
- **Substance Use Disorders**
- **The Psychiatric Interview**

PSYCHOTIC DISORDERS
A Practical Guide

Oliver Freudenreich, MD
Assistant Professor of Psychiatry
Harvard Medical School
Director, MGH First Episode and Early Psychosis Program
Massachusetts General Hospital
Boston, Massachusetts

Wolters Kluwer | Lippincott Williams & Wilkins
Health

Philadelphia · Baltimore · New York · London
Buenos Aires · Hong Kong · Sydney · Tokyo

01239824

Publisher: Charles W. Mitchell
Managing Editor: Sirkka Howes Bertling
Developmental Editor: Nancy Hoffmann
Project Manager: Jennifer Harper
Associate Director of Marketing: Adam Glazer
Manufacturing Coordinator: Kathleen Brown
Design Coordinator: Terry Mallon
Production Services: International Typesetting & Composition

© 2008 by Lippincott Williams & Wilkins, a Wolters Kluwer business
530 Walnut Street
Philadelphia, PA 19106 USA
LWW.com

Library of Congress Cataloging-in-Publication Data
Freudenreich, Oliver.
  Psychotic disorders : a practical guide / Oliver Freudenreich.
    p. ; cm.
  Includes bibliographical references and index.
  ISBN-13: 978-0-7817-8543-3
  ISBN-10: 0-7817-8543-X
1. Psychoses. 2. Mental illness. I. Title.
  [DNLM: 1. Schizophrenia—diagnosis. 2. Schizophrenia—therapy. 3. Antipsychotic Agents—therapeutic use. 4. Psychotic Disorders—diagnosis. 5. Psychotic Disorders—therapy. WM 203 F889p 2008]
  RC512.F7245 2008
  616.89—dc22

                                                                                    2007020743

DISCLAIMER
  Care has been taken to confirm the accuracy of the information presented and to describe generally accepted practices. However, the authors, editors, and publisher are not responsible for errors or omissions or for any consequences from application of the information in this book and make no warranty, expressed or implied, with respect to the currency, completeness, or accuracy of the contents of the publication. Application of this information in a particular situation remains the professional responsibility of the practitioner; the clinical treatments described and recommended may not be considered absolute and universal recommendations.
  The authors, editors, and publisher have exerted every effort to ensure that drug selection and dosage set forth in this text are in accordance with the current recommendations and practice at the time of publication. However, in view of ongoing research, changes in government regulations, and the constant flow of information relating to drug therapy and drug reactions, the reader is urged to check the package insert for each drug for any change in indications and dosage, and for added warnings and precautions. This is particularly important when the recommended agent is a new or infrequently employed drug.
  Some drugs and medical devices presented in this publication have Food and Drug Administration (FDA) clearance for limited use in restricted research settings. It is the responsibility of the health care provider to ascertain the FDA status of each drug or device planned for use in their clinical practice.
  To purchase additional copies of this book, call our customer service department at **(800) 638-3030** or fax orders to **(301) 223-2320.** International customers should call **(301) 223-2300.**
  Visit Lippincott Williams & Wilkins on the Internet: http://www.lww.com. Lippincott Williams & Wilkins customer service representatives are available from 8:30 am to 6:00 pm, EST.

10 9 8 7 6 5 4 3 2 1

3 0 JAN 2008

Meinem Vater

Contents

Foreword

This book is a rarity among books about schizophrenia. It is written by someone who spends the majority of his working life providing care to patients with schizophrenia. The authors of most books about schizophrenia spend their working lives writing grants and papers, and opining with their ilk at meetings on the basis of materials several steps distant from patient contact. Dr. Freudenreich is, at his core, a clinician, an astoundingly learned clinician who considers mitigating the effects of this disease on his patients' lives his most important purpose.

This book is about what is known *and* important. There is an immense literature on schizophrenia; thousands of new papers are published every year. History will show that more than 99% of what is published contributes nothing to the day-to-day care of patients with schizophrenia. Dr. Freudenreich is a voracious reader and careful curator of the schizophrenia literature. He provides for you in this book the quintessence (fifth distillate) of his scholarship. The material he has included has withstood repeated tests and challenges and has strong support. He tells you what you have to know and what you have to do to provide the best possible care for patients with schizophrenia.

If asked, almost all patients with schizophrenia deny that they are ill or need treatment. Yet, most come for their appointments and take their prescribed medications. When asked why they take their medications, having just denied a need for medications, they look surprised at the questioner's lack of sophistication and explain that "the doctor prescribed it." There is some common ground identified, if never reduced to words. There is some value applied in each patient's economy. Dr. Freudenreich's patients come to their appointments because he is interested in them. He understands their experiences that we, but not they, call psychopathology. He knows that they do not want to suffer side effects from their medications. He knows that they want the same things we want, ". . . something to do, and good people to do it with" (Hemingway). Dr. Freudenreich tries to hand them along on their ways toward these goals. He tells you in this book what you need to know to be able to do the same thing.

Joseph P. McEvoy, MD
John Umstead Hospital
Butner, North Carolina

Preface

"Well, doctor, tell me, exactly how many patients with this disease have you seen?," my psychiatric consultation fellowship director, George B. Murray, would invariably ask after I had once again self-assuredly presented to him in rounds a patient with a rare disease. Of course, I usually had to mumble "one, if you count this one." And George would invariably add, "So, in other words, you have not seen a lot of them?" His valid point, of course, was this: you can only know clinical medicine and psychiatry from seeing patients, many patients, that is, so you appreciate a disease in all its forms and shades, and phases and stages.

To learn about psychotic disorders, then, see as many patients with psychosis as you can and ask your teachers to help you understand what you see. In addition, read articles and books about psychosis to add understanding to your clinical experience. I hope this book is your starting point for your journey into the fascinating world of psychotic disorders.

This book is about clinical aspects of psychosis: how to recognize that somebody is psychotic, how to arrive at a clinical diagnosis that explains the psychosis, and how to treat it. Schizophrenia constitutes the bulk of patients with psychosis, and the bulk of this book is therefore dedicated to diagnosing and treating schizophrenia and related conditions. A perhaps unique bent for a psychiatric text is the emphasis on medical comorbidity, a partly iatrogenic scourge for many patients with schizophrenia, adding medical insult to psychiatric injury.

I think of this book as a *vade mecum* (Latin for "go with me"): a little manual to carry around in your pocket because it is useful, probably mainly for medical students, psychiatric residents, and other health care professionals who need to evaluate and treat a psychotic patient. This is not a textbook of psychosis, and you will find little discussion of neurobiology and pathophysiology.

To make the material come alive, clinical vignettes are dispersed throughout the text. All vignettes are based on real patients that I am currently treating but, to paraphrase Thomas Mann, consider the vignettes "descriptions of the way things never were but always are." Tips and key points are the clinical teaching pearls I use in my seminars or at the bedside, and should be taken with a grain of salt and not as absolutes. I included annotated recommendations for articles, books, and web sites for further study at the end of each chapter, as well as pocket cards for use in the clinic (covering emergencies, rating scales, and wellness) in the appendices.

The chapters are a condensation of my teaching of residents from the Harvard MGH-McLean program and the Boston University program; my research in the Massachusetts General Hospital Schizophrenia Program; and my clinical experience as an attending physician in an emergency department and a forensic inpatient unit, as a psychiatric consultant, and as an outpatient psychiatrist. I have even worked as an alienist in a state hospital (see History of Schizophrenia Care in the United States in the last chapter, if you are confused about what alienists do). So, I hope, my thoughts and recommendations are a blend of clinical wisdom and pragmatic advice that is informed by the literature.

If you have the time for feedback, simply e-mail me (ofreudenreich@partners.org). I welcome your comments about this *vade mecum*.

Oliver Freudenreich, M.D.

Acknowledgments

Nassir Ghaemi encouraged me to write this book and suggested my name to Charley Mitchell at Lippincott Williams & Wilkins, who trusted that I would produce a manuscript. Nancy Hoffmann, Sirkka Bertling, and Jennifer Harper turned the manuscript into a book. I am grateful to them, and to the editor of Practical Guides in Psychiatry, Daniel Carlat, who gave me the opportunity to contribute my favorite topic to his series.

What I wrote I could not have written without the mentorship of three individuals, in order of appearance in my professional life journey: Joseph McEvoy taught me most of what I know about the syndrome of schizophrenia. I will never forget my first few years in the country when I rounded with Joe at John Umstead Hospital in Butner, NC. Thank you, Joe, for those good years as your clinical research fellow. George Murray taught me general hospital psychiatry when I came to MGH to be one of his fellows on the psychiatric consultation service. George, your dictums and metaphors helped me appreciate the human condition and also see my own humanity. And Donald Goff, my current boss, taught me how to be an academic public-sector psychiatrist, if there is such a thing. Don, I am grateful that you continue to guide me through the thicket of clinical care, clinical research, and publishing.

My former co-fellows, now colleagues and always friends, John "Jack" Querques and Nick "Stavros" Kontos, helped me substantially with the book. Some teaching points are theirs, not mine. Without their friendship, and our own private think tank, Boston would be a much colder New England town.

My colleagues in the MGH Schizophrenia Program all dedicated their time and talents to critique individual chapters: Cori Cather, Eden Evins, Dave Henderson, Daphne Holt, Jen Park, and Tony Weiss. Our fellows, Constantin Tranulis and Ruth Barr, also edited chapters, as did Larry Park of MGH. I was lucky to have Raj Gandhi from the MGH HIV clinic always willing to help with "the medical stuff." Nassir Ghaemi was available to guide me through the process of writing a book whenever I needed him.

Stuart Schwartz at UMDNJ, as well as Janet Osterman and Dominic Ciraulo of Boston University, launched my teaching career. Unwittingly, the psychiatry residents at MGH-McLean and Boston University have helped create and fine-tune much of what is in this book. I thank them for their enthusiasm and keeping the special teacher–student relationship alive for me.

I am grateful to all the patients who trusted my judgment over the last decade or so, even if it was not their idea to see a psychiatrist. Through them, I have remained a student, and collectively they have given me more than I could ever have imagined.

Last, I thank my family for putting up with me "at the computer" instead of going to the ballet, throwing the football, or pushing the swing. Thank you, Catherine, Sheldon, and Sophie, respectively.

INTRODUCTION TO PSYCHOSIS

Psychotic Signs and Symptoms

Essential Concepts

- Descriptive psychopathology provides the building blocks for psychiatric diagnosis. It provides the language for observed behaviors and inner experiences.
- In a narrow sense, psychosis is operationally defined as the presence of delusions or hallucinations.
- Delusions are beliefs characterized by falsity, certainty, and incorrigibility.
- Delusions, hallucinations, formal thought disorder, and catatonia are considered positive symptoms.
- Knowing Schneiderian First-Rank Symptoms (FRS) is useful to screen for psychosis, not to make a specific diagnosis. Somebody who reports FRS is clearly actively psychotic.

> "Man sieht nur das, was man weiß."
> ("You only see what you know.")
> —*Johann Wolfgang von Goethe, 1749–1832*

Descriptive psychopathology is that branch of psychiatry that concerns itself with the precise definition of terms for clinical phenomena you might encounter when examining the mental state of a patient such as psychosis, the topic of this book. Descriptive psychopathology includes (a) observing behavior and (b) inquiring into the subjective experience of patients, with the goal not to explain, but to correctly identify their inner experience. The latter is a branch of descriptive psychopathology known as phenomenology. Karl Jaspers, who wrote the classic text on psychopathology, put it best: "Subjective symptoms cannot be perceived by the sense-organs, but have to be grasped by transferring oneself, so to say, into the other individual's psyche; that is, by empathy."

In this chapter, I describe the signs and symptoms to look for when deciding if somebody is experiencing psychosis. Read the descriptions, but then find teachers who will show you what the phenomena look like in real patients, to "feel the Mississippi mud between your toes," in the words of George Murray.

PSYCHOTIC SIGNS AND SYMPTOMS

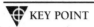 KEY POINT

In its most narrow conceptualization, psychosis is defined as the presence of delusions or clear-cut hallucinations, punctum. In broader definitions, formal thought disorder, behavioral disorganization, and catatonia are included in its definition. Psychotic symptoms are neither specific for any disorder nor even necessarily pathologic.

Conceptually, psychosis is "impaired reality testing," the famous "break from reality." Clinically, this is not terribly useful: How do you know when it is present? Attempts have been made to identify clinical signs and symptoms suggestive of psychosis, giving rise to the above operationalized definition of (narrowly defined) psychosis as delusions or hallucinations.

DELUSIONS

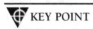 KEY POINT

For pragmatic, clinical purposes, delusions are fixed, false beliefs: Beliefs that are held with great conviction even in the face of overwhelming evidence to the contrary and are not shared by members of the patient's own culture or subculture.

You might think a core concept of psychiatry, the "basic characteristic of madness," as Karl Jaspers called delusions, is well understood. As it turns out, delusions defy easy understanding. Karl Jaspers identified three key characteristics of delusions: impossible content (falsity), held with conviction (certainty), and not susceptible to correction (incorrigibility). All three characteristics do not withstand closer scrutiny. Certainty in a delusional belief is frequently not absolute, but subject to doubt; and many patients can challenge and correct their assumptions (the basis for cognitive–behavioral treatment for psychosis). In contrast, we all hold certain beliefs dear to our heart with conviction and defend them against modification (e.g., scientific beliefs). Probably most problematic from a philosophical point of view is the assumption that "false" (impossible) ideas are somehow different from "unusual" or normal ideas. Often, delusions seem mere grotesque exacerbations of surrounding beliefs rather than "false." The impossible content problem leads to the inclusion of a reference group to determine the veracity of an idea by majority vote: if enough people (e.g., your church community) share your worldview, the idea is not considered delusional. I should say that, despite great theoretical problems, delusions are usually easy to spot in the clinic. The problem is reminiscent of defining pornography ("I know it when I see it," according to Supreme Court Justice Potter Stewart).

Once you have encountered a delusion, assess the following aspects:

- What is the delusion about? Delusions as a disorder of thought content are conveniently classified according to the dominant theme, e.g., delusions of grandeur, love, persecution, reference, control, and religious delusions. Table 1.1 lists eponyms of psychotic presentations.
- Is the delusion bizarre? This matters because, in current classification systems, bizarre delusions assume prominence: you can make the diagnosis of schizophrenia based on this one symptom alone (assuming the other criteria are fulfilled). If a delusion is considered bizarre, delusional disorder, in which delusions have to be nonbizarre, cannot be diagnosed. Kraepelin noted the delusions in dementia praecox "often show . . . an extraordinary, sometimes whole *nonsensical* stamp." Not even this is easy, however, and psychiatrists disagree when a delusion becomes bizarre (Spitzer et al., 1993). I would ask if an idea is (currently) physically possible to decide this matter.
- Is the delusion mood-congruent? Typically but not necessarily, the delusions of depression are morbid, those of mania grandiose.
- How pervasive is the delusion? Is it encapsulated within an otherwise intact personality, or are you dealing with a well-formed, systematized delusional system in which everything and everybody is connected to the delusion?
- How firmly entrenched is the delusion? Is doubt a possibility? Ask "Is it possible that you are wrong, that you are overinterpreting events and people's intentions?"

Although today often understood to mean persecuted, paranoia was the term Kraepelin originally used for conditions in which delusions were the only psychopathologic feature. The term is still used in that sense in "paranoid schizophrenia," a subtype of schizophrenia in which *any type* of delusion dominates the clinical presentation.

TABLE 1.1. Eponyms of Psychotic Presentations

Bell's mania Delirious mania: A severe form of excited mania in which the patient appears delirious (disoriented and with fever). Death from exhaustion can occur.

Capgra's phenomenon Delusion of doubles: A friend or relative has been replaced by an imposter (an exact double). Suspect organicity; it is often seen at some point in Alzheimer disease. The patient needs to be sent for neuropsychiatric testing and magnetic resonance imaging (MRI). Capgras is only one of several delusional misidentification syndromes. In the "illusion of Fregoli," a persecutor is seen in many people, as the persecutor is disguised and changes in appearance.

Charles Bonnet syndrome Vivid and complex visual (pseudo-) hallucinations that are the result of eye disease. The hallucinations are friendly, for example, little people sitting in living room. The patient needs to see an ophthalmologist.

De Clérambault syndrome Erotomania: Delusional conviction that somebody (usually a man of higher station) is in love with you (usually a female), despite virtually no contact. Can occur in its "pure," primary form or embedded in other psychiatric illnesses. Three stages: hope, resentment, overt hostility—the loved person is in danger in the third stage.

Ekbom's syndrome *Dermatozoenwahn.* Chronic tactile hallucinosis or delusional parasitosis: Patients imagine infestation with bugs, worms, insects. The patient often presents to dermatologist ("positive matchbox sign" with "trapped" evidence), but should see you. Make sure it is not amphetamine misuse.

Cotard's syndrome Characterized by nihilistic delusions: Patients believe they are dead; they believe they do not exist or that the world does not exist; that they have no heart; "I am being prepared for execution." It occurs in psychotic, depressive states.

Ganser syndrome Characterized by *"vorbeireden"*—talking past the point; giving approximate answers to simple questions; all answers are absurdly wrong, but just barely: 3 plus 3 is 7. A camel has five legs. Possibly malingering, maybe twilight state.

Korsakoff's psychosis A misnomer today, as no psychosis in the modern sense is present. It is the possible residual state of acute Wernicke encephalopathy. Patients cannot form new memories (anterograde amnesia) and confabulate. Try thiamine for treatment.

Kraepelin–Morel disease Rarely used eponym for schizophrenia.

Lhermitte's (peduncular) hallucinosis Vivid, colorful visual (pseudo-) hallucinations caused by a midbrain lesion.

(Continued)

TABLE 1.1. Eponyms of Psychotic Presentations (*continued*)

Münchhaüsen syndrome One of the factitious disorders. Patients seek admission to hospital, often with incredible stories (pseudologia fantastica). When patients are found wandering from hospital to hospital, they are known as "hospital hobos."

Othello syndrome Characterized by delusions of infidelity. Also occurs in alcoholics as morbid jealousy.

Overvalued Idea

The German psychiatrist Carl Wernicke (of Wernicke syndrome) used the term "overvalued idea" for people with a passionate attitude, also known as "fanatics" in lay terms. One important aspect of overvalued ideas is that they are shared with other people, making them potentially destructive. Remember that delusions, by contrast, are uniquely false ideas held by individuals and identified by others as erroneous. While most people would not jeopardize their careers or lives for overvalued ideas, some will (and are secretly regarded as heroes by those less inclined to fight for an idea). This is to say that it is not the idea itself but the reckless (toward oneself and others) pursuit that causes isolation and suffering. The term is problematic in that it makes it easy to label a person with differing opinions.

 TIP

The best way of getting patients to talk about delusions and delusionlike ideas is by taking a stance of curiosity and confusion, best exemplified by Peter Falk's LAPD Detective Columbo: "I am confused. On the one hand, you work for the CIA but then you are not getting a paycheck." With the Columbo technique, you challenge inconsistencies without appearing to doubt the patient's account of events.

HALLUCINATIONS

The French psychiatrist Jean-Étienne-Dominique Esquirol defined hallucination as a "percept without an object." Think of hallucinations as false perceptions (there is perception without an external object) in contrast to altered perceptions (e.g., illusions or sensory distortions where a real object is experienced as distorted).

Auditory hallucinations (AH) are frequent (although not obligatory) in schizophrenia. AH can be noises, but typical are "voices," more often unpleasant than pleasant. Three types of voices are so typical that they are used to diagnose schizophrenia (see below under Schneiderian First-Rank Symptoms). This does not mean that AH do not occur in other disorders or that hallucinations other than AH do not occur in schizophrenia. As a rule of thumb, visual hallucinations (VH) should make you suspicious of a delirium or dementia (Table 1.2). Descriptively, VH are either unformed (simple) or formed (complex). Olfactory hallucinations are typical for epileptic auras but can occur in schizophrenia, unfortunately for the patient usually as a fetid smell. Tactile hallucinations might suggest amphetamine use but also overlap with strange, bodily sensations, often of a sexual nature in schizophrenia (some use the mouthful "coenesthesia"). Some hallucinations occur only in certain situations: as hypnagogic or hypnopompic hallucinations during sleep–wake cycle transitions (consider narcolepsy) or as functional hallucinations (e.g., only when the shower is on or the air conditioner is humming).

 TIP

To evaluate hallucinations, ask directly: "Do you sometimes hear somebody talk, but to your surprise, nobody is around?" Then get specifics: "Where are the voices coming from? What are they saying? Are they insulting?" Do not miss command hallucinations: "Are they instructing you what to do?" Check for typical FRS hallucinations ("Shneiderian First Rank Symptoms" below).

TABLE 1.2. Visual Hallucinations in Nonpsychiatric Conditions

Delirium (often frightening)
Dementia
Toxic states and drug withdrawal
Organic lesions in visual pathways
Ocular pathology (e.g., Charles Bonnet syndrome)
Migraine
Epilepsy
Peduncular hallucinations from midbrain pathology

Pseudohallucinations

Some patients recognize that their hallucinations are "not real," or that they are "in their mind," that they could be their own thoughts. Some authors use "pseudohallucinations" to indicate the presence of insight into the pathology of the experience. A good example of pseudohallucinations is the visual hallucinations of the Charles Bonnet syndrome.

 TIP

With effective antipsychotic treatment, hallucinations take on the character of pseudohallucinations. Ask: "Point where you hear the voice" and "Is it possible that it is your own thoughts you are hearing?"

Hallucinosis

Hallucinosis describes a mental state characterized by hallucinations in a clear sensorium. Alcoholic hallucinosis and Lhermitte (peduncular) hallucinosis are well-recognized entities. Delusional interpretation of hallucinations is possible, albeit not prominent.

Schneiderian First-Rank Symptoms

Kurt Schneider, former chair of the department of psychiatry at Heidelberg University (my alma mater), lives on in his concept of "Schneiderian FRS." This is a list of originally 11 straightforward psychotic phenomena (Table 1.3) that are often encountered in schizophrenia and can be reliably identified. (I admit that there is some circular reasoning involved: Several FRS, because they are thought prototypical of schizophrenia, have become part of the definition of schizophrenia in current diagnostic systems.) They all capture the positive, paranoid–hallucinatory symptoms of psychosis.

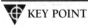 **KEY POINT**

None of the FRS is pathognomonic of schizophrenia; they lack specificity. You will hear about them, for example, from patients with delirium or a mood disorder. They are, however, very prevalent in schizophrenia and other nonschizophrenia psychotic disorders (Peralta and Cuesta, 1999). I use this fact to screen for psychosis by asking about FRS, not to make a specific diagnosis.

TABLE 1.3. List of Schneiderian First-Rank Symptoms

Primary Delusion (delusion is a sudden apophany or revelation)
   Delusional perception (an observation is misinterpreted)

Auditory Hallucinations
   Voices arguing
   Voices commenting (running commentary)
   Audible thoughts (thought echo, *Gedankenlautwerden*)

Delusions of Thought Interference
   Thought insertion/thought withdrawal/thought broadcasting

Delusions of Control ("Passivity experience, made experiences")
   Passivity of feelings (made feelings)
   Passivity of action (made volitional acts)
   Passivity of impulse (made impulses)
   Somatic passivity (made sensations)

Voices:
Get an exact description of the voices, which are usually insulting, talking to the patient in the third person ("He is such a loser"); second person voices are typical for the self-accusatory talk of the depressed person ("You are such a loser"). Are they talking among themselves about you (arguig voices)? Are they commenting on everything you do as you do it (running commentary)? Do people repeat aloud what you think (thought echo)?

Alien influence on thought, feeling, behavior:

Do you feel that your thoughts are not private? That people can read your thoughts?

Do you feel controlled by some force? That you are being hypnotized?

Do you feel as if your feelings or your actions or your thoughts are not your own?

Do you experience sensations such as being radiated? Being experimented on?

It is my impression that patients with schizophrenia who have one of the FRS have others as well (perhaps because all FRS are the expression of some basic failure to recognize thoughts, feeling, or behaviors as internally generated, patients instead attribute them to something coming or forced on from the outside; or, in Schneider's words, FRS are "a lowering of the barrier between the self and the surrounding world"). Note that the list of FRS includes delusions of thought and control that are considered bizarre (and thus eliminating delusional disorder as a differential diagnosis, when present). Often misunderstood is this: It is the experience that is delusional; there does not have to be a delusional explanatory system.

FORMAL THOUGHT DISORDER ("THOUGHT DISORDER")

Thinking can be disordered in two ways: by what patients say (problem with content, such as delusions), and how they say it (problem with form). If patients do not seem to make sense, not because of what they say but how they say it, a formal thought disorder (or disorder of thought process) might be present. Because we can only judge how somebody thinks by what the person says, this is also known as disorganized speech. In clear cases of disorganized thought, speech has lost its communicative function. In subtle cases, you might be initially impressed but come to conclude that many things the patient said were "pseudophilosophical."

 TIP

You need a speech sample to judge if a formal thought disorder is present: Let the patient talk and simply listen. Ask an "assay" question ("What do you think of European soccer?"), sit back and listen, then ask yourself how your patient is developing his or her ideas. If you cannot reconstruct your question or if it is unclear what is said (despite many words), a thought disorder might be present.

Before you diagnose a formal thought disorder, make sure you are not dealing with confusion (check orientation and attention) or aphasia (check if the patient can name, comprehend, and repeat).

In a thought disorder, thoughts are not properly associated, hence the overarching term looseness of associations (LOAs). Derailment or "knights move thinking" are other terms that describe the same phenomenon. Loose associations can be at the level of sentences or even within a sentence. In tangential speech each thought is connected to the next, but the overall goal is lost and never reached. If combined with an acceleration of speech, you have the flight of ideas of manic patients. In the extreme case of thought disorder, there is no connection between words and the patient becomes incoherent to the point of producing word salad.

In circumstantial speech, the goal of answering your question is not lost; the patient is merely adding unnecessary (and for a time-pressured physician) maddening detail. If you interrupt a long-winded, overinclusive patient, the patient will say "I know, I am getting to it," suggesting he or she has not lost track of the goal. This can be a personality quirk.

 TIP

In the mental status examination (MSE), I try to make a list of mild, moderate, or severe LOAs. I will also note neologisms (new words with meaning to the patient, e.g., to transchieve)—make sure you consult your dictionary before you note them; and non sequiturs (abrupt and unexpected statements that do not follow what was said. A patient might ask out of the blue: "Do you like pizza?"). I use the earthy term "rambling" to indicate LOAs that have a hard-to-interrupt, disinhibited quality.

BEHAVIORAL DISORGANIZATION AND CATATONIA

Peculiar motor behaviors can be clearly seen in old pictures and clinical descriptions of schizophrenia from the preneuroleptic era. Movements are not always easy to classify, and often convention replaces understanding. Common problems seen even in the absence of treatment with antipsychotics are mannerisms, stereotypies, grimacing, and spontaneous dyskinesias. Behavioral disorganization is a term used to indicate odd and bizarre behaviors like the ones just mentioned, but also other behaviors that are hard to put your finger on. These behaviors make your patient stand out, as social norms (or rules of common sense) are violated without obvious reason (i.e., patients are not trying to make a statement). Multilayered clothing in the summer, wearing a hardhat in the library, urinating or masturbating in public, and random shouting or laughter are examples of behavioral disorganization. Affect can be childlike, silly, or inappropriate to what you are discussing and prone to sudden shifts (you wonder if you are being belittled).

Catatonia can be viewed as an extreme form of bizarre motor behavior. Catatonic features are often missed because they are regarded as rare and hence not considered or examined for (Table 1.4). In a recent series of more than 100 consecutively

TABLE 1.4. Catatonia—Signs and Symptoms

Hypokinetic Phenomena

Catatonic stupor	Patient is immobile and unresponsive to environment
Catatonic mutism	Patient talks little or not at all
Catalepsy–posturing	Patient maintains a posture even if uncomfortable or imposed; if you try to move the patient, there can be some initial resistance, and the muscle tone feels like bending a wax candle (flexibilitas cerea, or waxy flexibility). Grimacing is seen if the face is affected, *Schnauzkrampf* if the "snout."
Staring	Patient stares straight ahead instead of looking around; blinks less.

Hyperkinetic Phenomena

Catatonic motor excitement	Motor activity without provocation and without purpose or goal
Stereotypies	Repetitive movements without goals; can be repetition of senseless movements (e.g., clapping, rocking) or of words (e.g., verbigeration or palilalia—repeating of phrases)
Mannerisms	Goal-directed, purposeful movements that appear odd, out of place, or exaggerated; e.g., saluting, unbuttoning; shaking hands in a stilted, awkward way; speaking with a fake accent
Echolalia and echopraxia	Two examples of echophenomena; patients repeat what they hear or what they observe (which gets in the way if they repeat the examiner's questions!).

Signs That Need to Be Elicited

Negativism	Without clear motive, patients resists your examination *Gegenhalten* (paratonia) is seen: The harder you try to move the patient, the harder the patient resists.

(Continued)

TABLE 1.4. (*continued*)

Automatic obedience	Patient is unable to resist instruction even if told to do something dangerous (e.g., "Stick out your tongue so I can pinch it with a needle"). *Mitgehen* is seen: Patients raises arm in response to light pressure even if instructed to resist.
Ambitendency	Patient hesitates and is stuck and indecisive to your conflicting instruction (e.g., stretching out greeting hand while telling patient "Don't shake my hand").

admitted psychiatric inpatients, 10% of patients displayed catatonic features (Chalasani et al., 2005). If you see one catatonic symptom, look for another; if you find two, you are probably dealing with catatonia.

 TIP

Consider a behavior bizarre if your patient fails the subway test (i.e., the crowd moves away from the patient because he or she is identified as having psychologic difficulties).

ADDITIONAL RESOURCES
Book

Sims ACP. *Symptoms in the mind: an introduction to descriptive psychopathology.* 3rd ed. London: Saunders; 2003.—Everything you need to know about psychopathology, written in clear language.

Article

Bar-El Y, Durst R, Katz G, et al. Jerusalem syndrome. *Br J Psychiatry.* 2000;176:86–90.—This article will get you curious about the complex relationship among normality, spirituality, religion, and psychosis.

Psychosis Interview

> "You can see a lot by observing."
> —*Yogi Berra, baseball Hall of Famer, 1972*

The great divide in psychiatric nosology between psychotic and nonpsychotic disorders makes identification of psychosis crucial for accurate differential diagnosis and proper treatment selection. Any psychiatric interview must, therefore, accomplish one thing: Ascertain with a reasonable degree of certainty that psychosis is either present or absent, both now and in the past. This chapter is not a comprehensive guide to the psychiatric interview but focuses on this aspect of the interview.

THE FIRST FEW MINUTES

Prepare for the patient encounter and review records that accompany the patient before you see him or her. Otherwise, you might never touch on the main reason for the patient's presentation and completely miss the boat.

Clearly introduce yourself. I always show patients my hospital ID tag (for the obvious problems with spelling and pronunciation of my name). Engage in some small talk on the way to your office ("Did you have trouble finding my office, finding parking?") to put patients at ease, if this is possible. After you sit down, an open-ended question that puts the ball in the patient's court is often the best way of starting: "What is the purpose of the visit with me?" or "How can I help you today?" To patients whose arms were twisted to come in, ask the question "Whose idea was it to come here today?" followed by "Does your family, the police have a point?" and "What is your side of the story?"

LOOKING FOR CURRENT PSYCHOSIS—HISTORY AND THE MENTAL STATUS EXAMINATION

The MSE (Table 2.1) can be considered the equivalent of the physical examination in medicine, with the organ under examination being the mind/brain. Just like the physical examination, the MSE is a cross-sectional record of signs of brain malfunction at the time of the examination (this is often done incorrectly, e.g. hallucinations heard earlier are recorded in the MSE—they should be noted in the history). In contrast to the physical examination, the MSE begins with the patient encounter and is interwoven with the history.

Data You Get from Observation

Observe your patient unobtrusively; I usually get patients from the waiting area myself so I can walk with them to my office. Is the patient laughing to himself or herself while waiting? Preoccupied and nervous? Paying attention to the surroundings?

TABLE 2.1. Suggested Format for the Mental Status Examination

Appearance, attitude, and behavior (including psychomotor abnormalities)
Affect and mood
Speech and thought process
Perception and thought content (psychosis, obsessions, SI, HI)
Sensorium and cognition (awareness and orientation; attention and memory; intelligence)
Insight and judgment

SI, suicidal ideation; HI, homicidal ideation.

What is he or she wearing? If somebody wears a T-shirt that says "Swabia Rules," ask about it!

Do not interrupt a patient who talks spontaneously, but simply listen. You need a good speech sample to judge speech and thought process. Interrupt politely yet firmly the rambling and disorganized patient who needs structure, once you have a first impression: "I have to interrupt you here and switch topics, if that's OK with you. We have not talked about your family." A patient's wallet and pockets can be windows to his or her functioning. Where does he or she put the prescriptions you wrote? How long does it take the patient to write down the new appointment date?

Data You Need to Inquire About

Although you can sometimes deduce your patient's inner experiences from behavior (e.g., patient is yelling back at voices), you usually have to inquire about them specifically.

 TIP

To screen for psychosis, I ask every patient two questions: "Have you ever had the sense that your thoughts were not private?" and "Have you noticed any coincidences lately?" The first question gets at audible thoughts and thought broadcasting or related experiences, the second at ideas or delusions of reference.

With patients in whom I suspect a psychotic illness, I always go through a complete list of psychotic symptoms and tell patients that I will ask them about experiences they might or might not have had. "If this has never been your experience, simply say no." Always ask specifically about strange bodily experiences patients cannot explain, as coenesthetic (somatic) hallucinations are often not reported spontaneously. Whereas bizarre delusions should become obvious to you during the interview, nonbizarre delusions can be missed, not because they are not mentioned but because they are not recognized as delusions. In the MSE, record "no delusions" (or "no obvious delusions," since you can never be absolutely sure), but do not write "patient denies delusions," which makes no sense.

You also need to ask about emotional experiences: "How would you describe your mood?"

Do not wait too long before you examine cognition. Early in the interview you should ask patients their birth date, the current date, and if they know where they are.

LOOKING FOR PAST PSYCHOSIS—PAST PSYCHIATRIC HISTORY

Collateral information is often crucial, as the patient might simply recall a "nervous breakdown," yet deny any history of psychotic symptoms. Some detective work and deductive reasoning are often required, judging by medications prescribed. I have encountered many patients with schizophrenia whose positive symptoms were remitted who simply denied a history psychosis: "I never heard voices."

 TIP

For past information, collateral information will often be more useful than patient recollection. Tracking down an old discharge summary that reveals the true meaning of "nervous breakdown" is time well spent.

COMMON MISTAKES IN THE ASSESSMENT OF PSYCHOSIS

- Accepting patients' description of their internal state. Somebody might say, "I get paranoid." Clarify what the patient means, summarize what you think you heard, and invite the patient to correct you. Always make sure you truly understand the patient and the patient understands you—the true meaning of phenomenology.
- Disregarding or overvaluing collateral information. It is a mistake to rely only on patients to rule out or rule in psychosis. On the other hand, make sure your patients are not being gaslighted (made to believe they cannot trust their senses and are going crazy—after the play *Gaslight*, by Patrick Hamilton).
- Disregarding limbic clues. If you feel threatened in any way, trust your limbic read of the situation and get out. Simply state, "Let me step out for a minute, I will be right back."
- Missing psychosis because of more prominent affective symptoms, particularly depression or irritability.

TABLE 2.2. Signs or Symptoms Suggestive of Psychosis

Marked reduction of interests and initiative
Marked social withdrawal
Aggression without purpose
Uncharacteristic self-neglect

Sometimes you will come away from the interview unsure whether the patient is psychotic. Psychosis can be intermittent or attenuated, or your patient may be unable to explain his or her experiences in sufficient detail to help you diagnostically. Assuring longitudinal follow-up in such cases will be the key intervention. At other times, if you think psychosis is possible (Table 2.2), but you are uncertain of the diagnosis, a drug trial can be offered. In any case, keep the diagnosis open. It is acceptable to put "undiagnosed" or "schizophrenia (working diagnosis)" in the chart.

PATIENTS UNABLE OR UNWILLING TO COOPERATE

Patient refuses to talk with you. Do not take it personally but try to figure out why. Is the patient afraid of something, is the patient paranoid, or is the patient angry? Tell the patient that it is in fact his or her choice to not talk with you. I sometimes summarize what I know, asking for input if this is correct. Point out that you are trying to help but that you will need some cooperation. Portray yourself as somebody sent in to help solve "the problem," merely a "cog in the machine" yourself.

Patient is very confused and makes little sense. Thought-disordered patients usually can contribute only limited information. This is the time to seriously consider a broad differential diagnosis, including dementia and a delirium. The main focus should be on the MSE and the physical examination. A neurologist might have to help to determine if an aphasia is present (e.g., if the onset of "thought disorder" was acute).

Patient is too psychiatrically ill to cooperate. A good example would be a volatile, manic patient or an irritable patient in a mixed episode. Once you have established the presence of a manic syndrome, start treatment. Do not waste time; often you accomplish the opposite of what you want, and the patient becomes more over-stimulated the more you ask. You can get more information later.

Patient is hostile or outright threatening. Abort the interview if you are uncomfortable; trust your limbic system, which is trying to warn you! You might have to treat in the face of insufficient information.

PATIENTS WHO MALINGER PSYCHOSIS

Some patients claim to be psychotic to avoid responsibility, get disability payments, or gain hospital admission. In any forensic context, the simulation of symptoms (or their exaggeration), technically known as malingering, is a real possibility.

CLINICAL VIGNETTE

A young homeless man presents to the emergency department on a snowy Boston night with a chief complaint of "the voices are telling me to walk into traffic." There is no formal thought disorder, no negative symptoms. He enjoys a sandwich and the company of other waiting patients while expecting admission.

One of the most common bogus complaints must be the solitary symptom of an auditory hallucination of the command type. In this setting and with no supporting evidence for psychosis beyond a single, stereotyped complaint, you should suspect malingering.

Here are some red flags that should raise your index of suspicion for malingered psychosis, particularly in the aforementioned settings:

- If very rare symptoms are reported
- If there are no supporting signs of schizophrenia except "voices"
- If the story keeps shifting during the evaluation process
- If the patient cannot identify anyone to give collateral information
- If there are many "I don't know" responses
- If patients give absurd answers to straightforward questions (because they falsely assume that psychotic patients are globally impaired)
- If you succeed in getting affirmative answers to absurd symptoms asked with a straight face (courtesy of Dr. Joseph P. McEvoy): "Do your bowel movements glow in the dark, do your teeth itch, or do you have pain behind your eyes when urinating (also known as retrobulbar mictalgia)?"
- If patients look sick with you but well on a smoke break
- If patients point out their "delusions" to you so you do not overlook them

TIP

Clearly document your assessment and choice of disposition. Be aware that you could be wrong *either way*. Even if you are sure that a patient malingers, always acknowledge uncertainty by saying "strong possibility of malingering," not "malingering, *punctum*."

ADDITIONAL RESOURCES

Book

Carlat DJ. *The psychiatric interview. A practical guide.* 2nd ed. Philadelphia, PA: Lippincott Williams & Wilkins; 2005.— From the same series as the book you are reading, a very practical guide to all aspects of the psychiatric interview.

DIAGNOSIS AND DIFFERENTIAL DIAGNOSIS OF PSYCHOSIS

3

Delirium

Essential Concepts

- Delirium is the clinical expression of an acutely failing brain, leading to disturbances of alertness and attention (also known as confusion). Delirium is often accompanied by agitation and psychosis.
- There is always at least one, sometimes several, medical causes for a delirium that need to be identified and treated.
- The treatment of choice for the delirium itself is antipsychotics, unless caused by sedative or alcohol withdrawal, in which case it is benzodiazepines.

"If you can't convince them, confuse them."
—*Harry S. Truman, 33rd US President, 1884–1972*

CLINICAL PRESENTATION

When the brain as an organ fails acutely from a wide variety of insults, a fairly stereotyped clinical syndrome, delirium, is the result. The onset of delirium is rather sudden, although an unspecific prodrome with anxiety and restlessness can predate the full-blown picture. One diagnostically useful hallmark of delirium is its fluctuation in severity over the course of the day. Delirium is fundamentally a disorder of attention: Patients are unable to pay attention, to shift attention, or to sustain attention. As attention is one of the basic brain functions that supports higher functions, other cognitive deficits are usually present. Patients are often unable to learn new information and appear puzzled, perplexed, and confused (hence the synonymous term "acute confusional state" for delirium). Patients are usually, *but not obligatory,* disoriented to time (often), place (sometimes), and person (only in severe cases); the key is the inability to attend. The level of consciousness can be altered in both directions, from hypervigilant to lethargic, stuporous, or comatose. Some patients are anxious, labile, and agitated (hyperactive delirium), others withdrawn (hypoactive delirium); most show a mixed pattern. Patients might be rambling or grossly incoherent. You should not expect to get a good history from a delirious patient. In addition, the sleep–wake cycle is disturbed and patients are awake at night and sleepy during the day.

Psychosis (delusions and hallucinations) is seen in 40% of deliria (Webster and Holroyd, 2000). The psychosis of delirium is characterized by fleeting, poorly formed delusions, often more a misinterpretation of the situation. Hallucinations are often visual; you may see patients picking at things. It is not always clear if you are dealing with misperceptions (illusions) and misinterpretations, or hallucinations and delusions. Table 3.1 presents a differential diagnosis of delirium.

DIAGNOSIS

Have a low threshold for suspecting a delirium in the right clinical setting. An elderly, hospitalized patient with new-onset psychosis has a delirium until proven otherwise, not late-onset schizophrenia. Any sudden change in clinical status is a red flag for the presence of a delirium. However, patients with known psychiatric disorders can have a superimposed delirium: A delirium can be superimposed on a manic patient who has not eaten or had anything to drink for days on his quest for the Holy Grail; a psychotic patient who is inadvertently overdosing on his benztropine because of confusion can be delirious. "Bad behavior" can stem from a subtly confused patient.

TABLE 3.1. **Differential Diagnosis of Delirium**

Dementia	Chronic onset, symptoms stable. Usually alert and able to attend. Immediate memory OK. Establish premorbid function with help of family members. Dementia is a risk factor for delirium.
Psychosis	Patients are alert and oriented with intact memory and attention. However, this can be difficult to assess in acute psychosis when patients are disorganized or uncooperative. Onset of psychotic illness is very rarely days but usually weeks. Psychosis can be part of delirium.
Depression	Can be confused with hypoactive delirium. Depressed patients can often participate in cognitive testing if you can get them motivated enough (persist when patient bemoans: "I can't do that.").

⬤ KEY POINT

A delirium *always* has a medical cause. Therefore, treatment begins with a search for medical etiologies. In many cases, not a single cause alone is responsible; (Table 3.2 presents etiologies of delirium). I like the term "acute brain failure" for delirium because it impresses a sense of urgency, as a delirium increases mortality.

Once you have suspected the presence of a delirium, identify its four cardinal features to make the diagnosis (these are taken from a widely used screening instrument, the Confusion Assessment Method, or CAM):

1. Acute onset with fluctuating course
2. Inattention (the patient was unable to focus on your questions or was easily distracted)
3. Disorganized thinking (the patient was rambling or hard to follow)
4. Altered level of consciousness (anything but alert)

Because alertness and attention have a "trickle-down" effect on other cognitive domains, the Mini-Mental State Examination (MMSE) supplemented with the clock-drawing test are excellent cognitive screens for bedside use (if patients can participate).

TABLE 3.2. Etiologies of Delirium

Withdrawal (alcohol, sedatives)
Intoxication (illicit drugs, medications, toxins)
Medical conditions
    Hypoxemia (from any cause, e.g., hypotension, anemia)
    Hypoglycemia
    Hypertensive encephalopathy
    Intracranial (stroke, encephalitis, tumor, trauma, bleeding, seizures)
    Infection (UTI, pneumonia, cellulitis, SBE)
    Metabolic (Wernicke's encephalopathy, hepatic encephalopathy, uremia, electrolyte abnormalities)
    Endocrine (thyroid, parathyroid, adrenal disease)

UTI, urinary tract infection; SBE, subacute bacterial endocarditis.

TIP

To briefly assess and follow a delirium longitudinally, a minimum bedside examination must note two things: the level of consciousness, and the degree to which attention is impaired. To gauge the latter, ask patients to recite the months of the year backwards (use days of the week if your patient has trouble doing the months).

A basic workup to identify the cause(s) is the next step (Table 3.3). The exact tests to order will depend on the clinical

TABLE 3.3. Initial Workup of Delirious Patients

History and chart review
Medication review
Vital signs
Physical and neurologic examination
Mental status examination with emphasis on cognition

Basic laboratory work-up:
   CBC with differential
   Glucose
   Chemistry profile, including calcium, magnesium, phosphate,
      and renal function
   Liver function tests (including ammonia level)
   TSH
   Serum drug levels (if applicable, e.g., digoxin, cyclosporine)
   Serum alcohol level
   Urine drug screen
   Urinalysis with C + S
   Electrocardiogram
   Chest X-ray

Ancillary tests:
   CT/MRI of brain if suspected intracranial process (MRI preferred
      unless intracranial hemorrhage suspected)
   LP if suspected brain infection
   EEG if suspected seizure activity (i.e., nonconvulsive status
      epilepticus or protracted postictal state)

Specific blood tests based on clinical situation (e.g., HIV test)

CBC, complete blood count; TSH, thyroid-stimulating hormone; CT, computed tomography, MRI, magnetic resonance imaging; LP, lumbar puncture; EEG, electroencephalogram; HIV, human immunodeficiency virus.

circumstances (i.e., which service consults you to help manage the delirium, as this will help determine the initial differential diagnosis of most likely offenders). As you are searching for an etiology, optimize the overall medical management.

 TIP

The electroencephalogram (EEG) of a delirious patient shows diffuse slowing (except for a delirium tremens where you see excess low-voltage beta activity). The EEG will assist in implementing your treatment plan if the medical team suspects the patient's behavior is willful. You cannot will an abnormal EEG!

Avoid these diagnostic mistakes:

- A delirium is not considered because the patient looked well at the morning evaluation. Serial examinations (and a chart review) are important as delirium fluctuates: Dr. Jekyll may look well at breakfast but still be Mr. Hyde at night. Without knowing a trend over several days, you cannot know if mental status is improving or merely waxing.
- A delirium is not considered because the patient has a history of schizophrenia and seems merely paranoid and thought disordered. The patient might not be paranoid but might not talk with you because of perplexity and confusion. A confused patient can be indistinguishable from a thought-disordered patient.
- An "underlying" psychiatric diagnosis is made in the presence of a delirium. You cannot make any psychiatric diagnosis until the delirium has cleared.
- Make sure you do not miss a delirium because you think the patient is catatonic. The treatment of catatonia with benzodiazepines can worsen a delirium.

TREATMENT

Antipsychotics are the mainstay of pharmacologic treatment for delirium unless the delirium is the result of alcohol/sedative withdrawal. Antipsychotics treat not only agitation and psychosis that can accompany any delirium but possibly the pathophysiology of delirium itself. For an acutely agitated patient after cardiac surgery, I tend to be conservative and use strategies with a proven track record and known toxicities (i.e., intravenous haloperidol). See EM CARD IV haloperidol (Appendix A) for guidance about the use of haloperidol.

One advantage of haloperidol is that it can be given orally, intramuscularly (IM)?, IV, and as a drip. Curiously enough, when given IV at large doses, immediate motor side effects are benign (Menza et al., 1987). In less acute situations, low-dose, second-generation antipsychotics (e.g., risperidone 0.25 to 1 mg bid, olanzapine 2.5 to 5 bid, or quetiapine 25 to 50 bid) have largely supplanted the use of haloperidol. Other pharmacologic approaches (e.g., anticholinesterase inhibitors) have some support in the literature but cannot substitute for antipsychotics if the clinical situation calls for them. I would argue that IV haloperidol represents the safest and most effective approach to treat *any* delirium unless there are specific contraindications to its use.

Avoid these common mistakes when you are treating a delirium:

- Treatment is not instituted immediately and/or not followed-up. Be prepared to help implement and monitor your clinical plan closely.
- Pharmacotherapy becomes confusing if you use several agents to treat agitation. I would pick one agent and stick with it. In particular, avoid benzodiazepines if you can, so as not to worsen confusion (except in alcohol or sedative withdrawal).

 TIP

I try to discontinue antipsychotics used to treat a delirium before a patient goes to rehabilitation or home to minimize the risk of tardive dyskinesia (TD) and neuroleptic malignant syndrome (NMS), although with short hospital stays this might not always be possible. In older patients, the TD risk even from short-term exposure (e.g., a few weeks) is very high.

Nonpharmacologic measures to prevent a delirium should be implemented (Inouye et al., 1999). Avoid excessive stimulation and provide a structured and safe environment (e.g., large clock, pictures of family members, remove dangerous items) for the patient at risk for delirium. Get patients their eyeglasses and hearing aids, so they are not sensory deprived. However, these measures are ancillary and no substitute for the proper pharmacologic treatment, once a delirium has developed. Optimal pharmacotherapy will decrease the need for physical restraints, which may even increase agitation as a confused patient tries to remove them.

ADDITIONAL RESOURCES

Book Chapter

Cassem NH, Murray GM, Lafayette JM, et al. Delirious patients. In: Stern TA, Fricchione GL, Cassem NH, et al. eds. *Massachusetts General Hospital handbook of general hospital psychiatry*. 5th ed. Philadelphia: Mosby; 2004:119–134.—From my department's book on general hospital psychiatry.

Article

Hall W, Zador D. The alcohol withdrawal syndrome. *Lancet.* 1997;349:1897–1900.—Still the best on alcohol withdrawal, which I did not cover in this chapter.

Drug-Induced Psychosis

Essential Concepts
- Some drugs of abuse cause psychosis during intoxication (or during withdrawal in the case of alcohol or sedative–hypnotics). Prolonged psychosis is typical for phenylcyclohexylpiperidine (PCP) and methamphetamines.
- History of drug ingestion supported by urine drug testing and resolution of symptoms in a manner characteristic for the drug suggests a drug-induced psychosis.
- Chronic alcoholism can cause chronic psychosis in the form of alcoholic hallucinosis and delusional jealousy (Othello syndrome).
- Cannabis increases the risk of eventually being diagnosed with schizophrenia sixfold. It is unclear if cannabis triggers an illness that would have never occurred or merely pushes the onset into earlier ages.
- Stimulants and hallucinogens predictably cause a short-lived, drug-induced psychosis (except for methamphetamine psychosis, which can last weeks).
- PCP can cause a severe, agitated psychosis lasting many days.

> "Drugs are a bet with your mind."
> —*Jim Morrison, The Doors, 1943–1971*

Many drugs can cause psychosis (delusions and/or hallucinations) in a clear sensorium (i.e., in the absence of a delirium). This is true not only for legal drugs (e.g., alcohol) or illegal drugs but also for prescribed medications (e.g., steroids or digoxin), herbal medications, and over-the-counter medications. In this chapter, I discuss patients who present to the emergency department (ED) with drug-induced psychosis. For a discussion of drug abuse in schizophrenia, see the chapter on dual diagnosis (Chapter 23).

DIAGNOSIS OF DRUG-INDUCED PSYCHOSIS

Some drugs predictably induce psychosis in most individuals after single use: PCP and lysergic acid diethylamide (LSD) are examples. Some drugs do so only in a small minority of patients (cannabis), or after prolonged use (cocaine). The major drugs that cause psychosis during withdrawal are alcohol and the sedative–hypnotics (barbiturates and benzodiazepines), as well as one of the club drugs, γ-hydroxybutyrate (GHB) (Table 4.1). Opiates as a rule of thumb are not associated with psychosis, although exceptions exist.

The diagnosis of drug-induced psychosis is somewhat complex, and one must look at history of drug use, symptoms, and results of urine drug testing. Ideally, a 4-week period of abstinence is necessary to judge if psychosis resolves in a time course consistent with the drug. Unfortunately, the necessary abstinence period is frequently not achieved, and you are left wondering how much psychosis is fueled by intermittent, low-grade drug use.

History of Drug Use

The history of drug use might be unavailable or incomplete. Patients themselves might not know what they ingested, or whether they were taking adulterated drugs (e.g., cannabis with PCP). Therefore, urine drug testing is mandatory even in cases in which a specific drug or no drug use is reported.

TABLE 4.1. Drug-Induced Psychosis

	During Intoxication	During Withdrawal	Prolonged
Alcohol	Yes	Yes	Yes
Sedatives	Yes	Yes	Yes
Cannabis	Yes	No	Not usually
Stimulants	Yes	No	Yes (methamphetamine)
Hallucinogens	Yes	No	Not usually
PCP	Yes	No	Yes
Opiates	Not usually	Not usually	Not usually

TIP

The drug culture has its own lingo. Don't play it cool; ask if you don't know. I always ask what patients mean if they use a drug name (those are not tightly regulated and patients might use the names differently from you).

Urine Drug Testing

Urine for drug testing should be obtained routinely in psychotic patients who present to the ED. This rule applies to new-onset psychosis but also to patients with established schizophrenia, as comorbid drug use is so common (but not recognized). However, there are limitations to what drug testing can accomplish you can only detect what you test for. Most urine drug screens (UDS) contain the standard "National Institute on Drug Abuse (NIDA) 5": cocaine, amphetamines, cannabis, opiates, and PCP, supplemented by benzodiazepines and barbiturates. Note that drugs that interest us in the context of psychosis but are not tested for include LSD, hallucinogens, and so-called club drugs. If a drug test is negative, the timing between ingestion and testing might simply have been too long, and the urine drug level fell below the detection limit of the assay. Even if a drug test is positive, this does not establish that the drug is in fact responsible for the clinical state.

Except for a serum alcohol level, serum drug testing is rarely useful in the ED unless results are immediately available. Serum cocaine levels can be useful because positive results indicate recent (within a few hours) use. Other tests, such as benzodiazepine levels, might still be useful for diagnostic purposes later on and you might consider saving a tube of blood.

TREATMENT OF DRUG-INDUCED PSYCHOSIS

Deciding how best to treat a self-limited drug-induced psychosis is difficult, as antipsychotics pose some risks (e.g., causing acute dystonic reactions if patients have used cocaine; van Harten et al., 1998). Consider using benzodiazepines alone as your initial treatment if you think psychosis is drug induced, mild, and you expect quick improvement (e.g., uncomplicated cocaine intoxication); but do not hesitate to use antipsychotics if benzodiazepines alone prove insufficient. Obviously, you recommend substance-use treatment and cessation of substance use.

SPECIFIC SUBSTANCES OF ABUSE

Alcohol and Sedative–Hypnotics

Several psychotic disorders can occur in alcoholics. Alcohol (and sedative–hypnotics) can cause psychosis during intoxication (rare), during withdrawal, or during delirium tremens. In chronic alcoholics, more persistent psychosis in the form of alcoholic hallucinosis, pathologic jealousy (Othello syndrome), or paranoia can develop.

CLINICAL VIGNETTE

A man in his forties who had been a heavy drinker for decades was admitted to a psychiatric inpatient unit after detoxification because of persecutory delusions and persistent auditory hallucinations. He had brought with him tapes he had made to capture the very prominent derogatory voices. No antipsychotics were administered, and his hallucinations resolved completely within a week. Two weeks after admission, we listened to the tapes together. He agreed that there was nothing recorded but maintained: "I know that the voices are on there because I heard them and recorded them."

This case of alcoholic hallucinosis illustrates that severe alcoholism can result in psychosis. Antipsychotics should be withheld to see if hallucinations resolve during a period of sobriety. It is important not to confuse ongoing psychosis with memories of the deluded state; in this case, the patient was unable to recognize his past experiences as the result of psychosis but he was not actively psychotic. In any alcoholic, treat nutritional deficiencies with thiamine to prevent Wernicke–Korsakoff's syndrome.

Cannabis

Cannabis ("weed," "reefer") use is widespread and often considered fairly innocuous. Apart from the obvious potential for legal problems, however, there has been the vexing possibility that cannabis is psychotogenic for a small group of biologically predisposed patients. In one study, the frequent use of cannabis (more than 50 times) assessed at time of conscription into military service increased the risk for developing schizophrenia in 15-year follow-up by sixfold (Andreasson et al., 1987). Put differently, cannabis is one of the strongest risk factors known for schizophrenia!

 TIP

Not that anyone should take cannabis, but anyone with a family history of psychosis or personal history of unusual experiences from experimentation with cannabis should abstain.

Stimulants: Cocaine and Amphetamines, Prescription Stimulants

Amphetamines are sold legally as prescription stimulants, and produced illegally as methamphetamine (speed, crystal meth) and the designer club drug methylenedioxymethamphetamine (MDMA [Ecstasy or "Adam"]; for more information, see the hallucinogen section), among others.

Stimulants can cause psychosis in normal people if taken at a high enough dose. Judging by psychopathology alone, it is impossible to distinguish a drug-induced stimulant psychosis from primary schizophrenia. Harris and Batki (2000) carefully characterized 19 patients with stimulant-induced psychosis: 95% had bizarre delusions, 64% had Schneiderian First-Rank Symptoms, and 26% had substantial negative symptoms. Cocaine has a short half-life and psychosis is short-lived. In patients with a decade or so of cocaine use, cocaine-induced psychosis can last longer and is accompanied by choreoathetoid motor abnormalities ("crack dancing"). This is important to know: If somebody presents to the ED with clear psychosis several hours after cocaine use, he or she is probably vulnerable and/or severely addicted. Unfortunately, in some locales, this simple rule of thumb is no longer useful: If methamphetamine is used, drug-induced psychosis can last days or even weeks. In college populations, the misuse of prescription stimulants is rampant and psychosis from high-dose use is possible.

In stimulant-induced psychosis, you might have to use antipsychotics if psychosis does not resolve in a few hours or if psychosis is severe enough to impair judgment (e.g., paranoia leading patients to feel they need to defend themselves).

 TIP

The presence of *formication* (the tactile hallucination that insects are crawling on the body or under the skin) should alert you to the possibility of cocaine use ("cocaine bugs") or methamphetamine use ("meth mites"). Look for skin excoriations from picking in this drug-induced form of delusional parasitosis. Other possibilities include delirium tremens or benzodiazepine withdrawal.

LSD and Hallucinogens

Although many hallucinogens can be found naturally in plants (e.g., morning glory seeds or "magic" mushrooms containing psilocybin and psilocin, mescaline from the peyote cactus) and have been used in many cultures, hallucinogen use took off with the discovery of the prototypical hallucinogen, LSD (German for *Lysergsäuredietylamid*) by the Swiss chemist Albert Hofmann of Ciba in 1943. While LSD is safe medically (not psychiatrically), hallucinogens that are derived from amphetamines (and are sometimes classified with amphetamines), e.g., MDMA, can lead to renal failure, seizures, and death. Some plant-derived hallucinogens, e.g., Jimson weed, can cause anticholinergic toxicity.

LSD is the most potent hallucinogen. A dose of only 20 μg has a marked effect. LSD trips last 12 hours, with another 12 hours recovering. A typical "acid trip" has prominent visual distortions: colors, shapes are altered; synesthesias (most often as seeing sounds); out-of-body experiences. This state of altered perception is usually accompanied by euphoria, but "bad trips" with panic can occur.

Most intoxications with hallucinogens are short lived, usually measured in hours or a few days at the most. One of the pioneers in LSD research, Henry David Abraham, has written that LSD trips can be good, bad, or permanent. Permanent damage in the form of flashbacks (the modern term is hallucinogen persisting perception disorder or HPPD) is well accepted. In susceptible individuals, even one-time use of LSD is feared to be able to trigger schizophrenia. The clinical picture of psychosis in "acid heads" is not distinguishable from schizophrenia, although auditory hallucinations are rare. Expect to discuss themes of cosmic peace and altered reality.

PCP and Ketamine

PCP ("angel dust") and its analogue, ketamine ("Special K") deserve a separate entry, as they produce a model psychosis that is indistinguishable from schizophrenia. Originally developed as dissociative anesthetics, these agents were found to induce psychosis in patients who received them for anesthesia.

PCP is often smoked and mixed with cannabis, frequently sold as something else, or used to adulterate other drugs. PCP can cause severe psychosis and severe violence. Medical complications are possible as PCP is catecholaminergic (hyperthermia and seizures). A neurologic sign, nystagmus, is fairly specific. Because PCP is lipophilic, it is released over days, leading to prolonged psychosis lasting many days. Ketamine has a much shorter duration of action and is one of the club drugs. It is usually eaten, smoked, snorted, or injected. Note that while PCP is often included in urine drug tests and can be detected for many days after use, ketamine is not revealed by the PCP assay.

ADDITIONAL RESOURCES

Web Sites

http://www.nida.nih.gov/.—The National Institute on Drug Abuse (NIDA) Web site.
http://www.clubdrugs.org/.—The NIDA Web site dedicated to club drugs.

5 Secondary Schizophrenia

Essential Concepts

- Before diagnosing primary schizophrenia, you must rule out secondary schizophrenia (i.e., schizophrenic symptoms are secondary to a nonpsychiatric medical disorder, either from a systemic disorder that affects the brain or from demonstrable neuropathology in the brain).
- A significant minority of patients with first-episode schizophrenia, around 5%, will have an identifiable, medical etiology of their psychosis.
- A wide variety of medical/neurologic disorders and some toxins are associated with psychosis.
- Their diagnoses without ancillary signs and symptoms require a combination of screening, a high index of suspicion, and clinical follow-up.
- Even if psychosis is the result of identifiable pathology, treatment with an antipsychotic in addition to treating the underlying disorder is often necessary.

"From error to error one discovers the entire truth."
—*Sigmund Freud, 1856–1939*

Many medical disorders can potentially mimic schizophrenia. For those schizophrenia like psychoses that are the result of medical illness, I follow the suggestion of Spitzer et al. (1992) to abandon the old term, "organic mental disorder," and use "secondary schizophrenia" instead. The distinction between primary and secondary disorders is familiar to most physicians, and it does not imply that schizophrenia is not brain based (a wrong conclusion fostered by calling it a "functional" disorder). This leaves four possibilities when faced with schizophrenic symptoms: primary schizophrenia; secondary schizophrenia (i.e., symptoms are secondary to a nonpsychiatric medical disorder, either a systemic disorder that affects the brain or demonstrable neuropathology in the brain); substance-induced psychosis (see previous chapter); and psychiatric disorders with psychotic symptoms (see following chapter). For brevity's sake, I still occasionally use the adjective "organic" to indicate nonpsychiatric causes.

CLINICAL VIGNETTE

A young man developed a textbook case of paranoid psychosis. During the routine workup for first-episode psychosis, a pituitary tumor was detected by magnetic resonance imaging (MRI) and partially resected. The patient now receives maintenance treatment for schizophrenia, as well as a dopamine agonist to reduce prolactin levels.

This case exemplifies the occasional scenario of an incidental discovery of a medical condition during the workup for first-episode psychosis. You will need to judge if the discovered medical condition is etiologically related to the psychosis, etiologically unrelated yet important for management, or etiologically unrelated and not important for management. In this case, the finding is etiologically unrelated to schizophrenia but complicates the management of schizophrenia (treatment with a dopamine agonist).

Johnstone et al. (1987) found organic disease (judged to be etiologically relevant for the psychiatric presentation) in 15 out of 268 (less than 6%) patients with first-episode schizophrenia. Specific conditions identified were syphilis, sarcoidosis, alcohol excess, drug abuse, lung cancer, autoimmune multisystem disease, cerebral cysticercosis, thyroid disease, and previous head injury.

 TIP

A multiaxial approach (i.e., simply listing schizophrenia and medical conditions without making assumptions about their relationship) is often most appropriate unless the psychosis is clearly the result of the medical disorder. If you think that controlling the medical disorder will eventually resolve the psychosis, you are probably dealing with a secondary psychosis.

DIAGNOSIS

There is no generally agreed-upon workup that every patient with psychosis must have. Follow these principles to exclude secondary schizophrenia:

- Order a screening test battery to exclude common and a few selected yet very treatable disorders (Table 5.1).
- An MRI will provide reassurance that a silent brain tumor (e.g., frontal lobe meningioma) is not missed, although the clinical yield of ordering an MRI will be low (Lubman et al., 2002). Expect to detect the mostly innocuous, incidental MRI abnormalities seen in 20% of the normal population (Katzman et al., 1999).
- Electroencephalograms (EEGs) can be difficult to interpret since almost half of patients with first-episode schizophrenia will have EEG abnormalities of unclear significance (Manchanda et al., 2005). Moreover, a normal EEG does not exclude medial brain abnormalities and interictal psychosis (schizophrenia like psychosis of epilepsy; see below under Neurologic Conditions).
- More tests are not necessarily better: Indiscriminate screening for rare disorders is inadvisable because of false-positive and false-negative test results. Order specific tests to rule in or out a disorder you suspect clinically.

TABLE 5.1. Initial Workup for First-Episode Schizophrenia[a]

Imaging studies[b]	*Laboratory studies (contd.)*
• MRI to rule out demyelinating disease, brain tumor (e.g., meningioma)	• Liver function tests
	• Erythrocyte sedimentation rate (ESR)
EEG[c]	• Antinuclear antibodies
Laboratory studies	• Ceruloplasmin
• Complete blood count	• HIV screening[c]
• Electrolytes	• FTA-Abs for syphilis (*RPR not sufficient*)
• BUN/creatinine	• Vitamin B_{12} and folate
• Glucose	• Urinalysis
• Calcium and phosphorus	• Urine drug screen
• TSH	

BUN blood urea nitrogen, *CXR* chest X-ray

[a]This list of tests is not exhaustive but represents merely one possible initial workup. Other tests should be considered if the clinical history and the clinical picture suggest that they might be useful diagnostically (e.g., EEG, CXR, lumbar puncture, karyotype).

[b]Controversial, as yield is low.

[c]Recommended as part of routine care for psychotic patients (Branson et al., 2006).

- Order the correct tests; for example, to exclude neurosyphilis, your patient needs to have the highly sensitive serum fluorescent treponemal antibody absorption test (FTA-Abs) and a lumbar puncture (LP), not the commonly ordered rapid plasma reagin (RPR).
- In poorly responsive psychosis, expand your search to exclude a paraneoplastic syndrome, epilepsy, and sarcoidosis.
- Expand your search for medical etiologies in atypical presentations (atypical with regard to age or symptoms).

 TIP

Longitudinal follow-up by the same person is probably the best safeguard against missing secondary schizophrenia, assuming that the medical disease "declares itself." Thus, any change in symptoms or new symptoms should lead you to revisit your initial impression.

SECONDARY SCHIZOPHRENIAS

Genetic Disorders

Several genetic syndromes have an increased risk for schizophrenia, particularly Klinefelter's syndrome, fragile X syndrome, and velo-cardio-facial syndrome (VCFS). VCFS, which stems from a deletion on the long arm of chromosome 22 (22q11), is strongly associated with schizophrenia like presentations, possibly in up to 25% of VCFS cases (Murphy et al., 1999).

 TIP

Currently, genetic testing is not recommended for patients with psychosis unless there is the clinical suspicion that a syndrome is present (e.g., family history of Huntington's disease). Even if there is no treatment, making a syndromal diagnosis is important for counseling and to look for other syndromal features (e.g., treatable cardiac problems that might be part of a syndrome).

Endocrine Disorders

One of the easiest-to-correct endocrine conditions associated with psychosis is hypoglycemia. Screen for thyroid disorders with a thyroid-stimulating hormone test (TSH), to exclude both hyperthyroidism and hypothyroidism (myxedema madness). In addition, consider Addison's disease, Cushing's disease, and hyperparathyroidism, as well as hypoparathyroidism.

Metabolic Disorders

Many inborn errors of childhood include psychosis in the list of possible symptoms. Almost all are diagnosed during childhood but atypical, adult onset is possible. Only acute intermittent porphyria is sufficiently common that you should suspect it if abdominal pain and peripheral motor neuropathy are present in a patient with psychosis.

 TIP

It is probably almost impossible to diagnose a rare presentation (psychosis alone) of a rare disorder (metabolic disorder) that presents at an atypical age (in adulthood). You need other clues and a high index of suspicion that would suggest a metabolic disorder.

Autoimmune Disorder

The most important disorder to consider is systemic lupus erythematosus (SLE). In the case of SLE, treatment with steroids greatly complicates diagnostic issues. Rarely, paraneoplastic syndromes or myasthenia gravis can cause psychosis.

Narcolepsy

The hypnagogic hallucinations that are part of the narcolepsy tetrad (in addition to cataplexy, sleep paralysis, and excessive daytime sleepiness) can lead to a mistaken diagnosis of schizophrenia. In one series of state hospital patients diagnosed with schizophrenia, 7% were found to suffer from narcolepsy (Douglass et al., 1991). In some, psychosis is probably related to the treatment of narcolepsy with stimulants.

 TIP

Consider a sleep study and human leukocyte antigen (HLA)-typing if psychosis is only related to sleep–wake transitions, even in the absence of other symptoms of narcolepsy.

Neurologic Conditions

Stroke. Poststroke psychosis is a possible but rare complication of stroke. To complicate matters, in many cases seizures obfuscate the picture and might be related to the emergence of psychosis. Peduncular hallucinosis is a syndrome of vivid, colorful formed visual hallucinations, often of animals (e.g., of a parrot in full plumage), with localizing value as focal lesions of the midbrain cause them, hence peduncular.

Seizures. Epilepsy and psychosis share a long history (Sachdev, 1998), and many psychiatrists have noted that there seems to be a higher prevalence of schizophrenia in patients with epilepsy (seizures leading to psychosis) but also an antagonism between the two conditions (seizures treating psychosis, leading to the development of electroconvulsive therapy, or ECT). Particularly in temporal lobe epilepsy, neurodevelopmental lesions are common. Psychosis following seizures (postictal psychosis) typically emerges within a day after the seizure and can last a few weeks or even months, and can resolve or with time develop into a more chronic condition. The interictal schizophrenia like psychosis of epilepsy does not emerge until a decade or more after seizures first occur, suggesting that epilepsy is a risk factor for this type of psychosis. Many patients with epilepsy display other psychiatric symptoms, including significant negative symptoms (Getz et al., 2002).

Demyelinating diseases. It is interesting that the most common demyelinating disease, multiple sclerosis, does not usually cause psychosis. Other, rare disorders affecting white matter are more likely to cause psychosis (i.e., the leukodystrophies: metachromatic leukodystrophy, X-linked adrenoleukodystrophy, and Marchiava–Bignami disease).

Basal ganglia disorders. In this category, Huntington's, Wilson's and Parkinson's disease are thought to be associated with psychosis. Psychosis can precede motor symptoms in Huntington's disease, but the diagnosis should become clear with the emergence of motor symptoms. Although screening for Wilson's disease (because it is treatable) is usually suggested as part of a psychosis workup, there is doubt in the literature that Wilson's disease can in fact present with schizophrenia like psychosis alone (Dening and Berrios, 1989). The psychosis of Parkinson's disease is characterized by visual hallucinations, often attributed to antiparkinsonian medications but more recently linked to rapid eye movement (REM) sleep behavior disorder (RBD).

TIP

Any time you are dealing with extreme sensitivity to antipsychotics or the early development of a movement disorder (mistakenly attributed to antipsychotics as tardive dyskinesia), consider a neurology consult to exclude neurologic disease.

History of head injury. Significant head injury, including the temporal lobes, is a risk factor for the eventual development of psychosis. There is a substantial lag time of several years between the head injury and the emergence of psychosis.

Dementias. Dementias are commonly accompanied by behavioral problems such as agitation, depression, and psychosis. Psychosis is seen in the most common form of dementia, Alzheimer's dementia, particularly in later disease stages (Craig et al., 2005). In Lewy body dementia (LBD), recurrent and well-formed visual hallucinations are a core diagnostic feature of the disease (McKeith et al., 2005). Very poor tolerability of antipsychotics (prescribed for the hallucinations) is a clinical tip-off. Neuropsychiatric symptoms greatly complicate dementia management and are often the proverbial straw that breaks the camel's back, leading to institutionalization.

Brain tumors. The major concern is missing frontal lobe tumors that are "silent"; i.e., the neurologic examination is normal. Meningiomas are treatable! Other space-occupying lesions have been implicated in psychosis (e.g., cerebrovascular malformations involving temporal lobes, brain abscess, or cysts, cerebrovascular malformations involving temporal lobes

Vitamin Deficiencies

Pernicious anemia must be ruled out in every patient (by checking vitamin B_{12} level), as psychosis can predate neurologic symptoms. Pellagra (niacin deficiency) is now very rare in the United States but used to be the prototype of a reversible psychosis from a nutritional deficiency. Look for the four Ds—dementia, dermatitis, and diarrhea (and death as the fourth one)—and for stomatitis and glossitis. Very rarely, vitamin A, vitamin D, and zinc deficiencies have been associated with psychosis.

Infections

Infections are important, often treatable causes of psychosis. The exact pathogens will vary, depending on region and immune status; consider tuberculosis, cerebral malaria, toxoplasmosis, and neurocysticercosis, when appropriate. In the United States, the most important infections to rule out are herpes simplex encephalitis, followed by neurosyphilis and human immunodeficiency virus (HIV). In a case series of neurosyphilis in the antibiotic era, 82 of 161 (51%) patients with confirmed neurosyphilis had only neuropsychiatric symptoms, mostly in the form of slowly developing dementia with episodes of delirium. Even though HIV was not identified as a cause of psychosis in a military sample of more than 200 recruits admitted for a first psychotic episode, HIV can present with psychosis. Neuroborreliosis (Lyme disease) is often listed as a cause of psychosis, although evidence for direct causation is lacking.

Toxins

Psychosis that is caused by environmental toxins requires a high index of suspicion. Take into account patients' living situations and occupations to make a judgment if they could be poisoned by any of the following toxins: carbon monoxide, heavy metals (arsenic, manganese, mercury, thallium), or organophosphates.

TREATMENT

The best treatment for secondary psychosis is the treatment of the underlying disorder *and concomitant treatment of psychosis.* Only in mild cases, when a rapid correction of the medical problem and rapid resolution of psychosis are expected, should you delay antipsychotic treatment. Often, you will still have to treat the psychosis symptomatically with an antipsychotic, as resolution of psychosis might lag behind greatly (or the underlying disorder is not treatable). Note that the dosing guidelines for antipsychotics are based on treating schizophrenia, and patients with psychosis from medical causes are generally neuroleptic-naïve and very sensitive to extrapyramidal side effects. In some disorders that affect basal ganglia (e.g., Parkinson's disease or HIV disease), this can cause major difficulties with finding a tolerable regimen. To minimize the risk for tardive dyskinesia, limit the exposure to antipsychotics in medical patients.

Antipsychotics are problematic for older patients with dementia-related psychosis. First-generation antipsychotics carry a very high risk of tardive dyskinesia for geriatric patients. Unfortunately, second-generation antipsychotics (SGAs) have just been shown to be neither particularly effective nor well tolerated. In the Clinical Antipsychotic Trials of Intervention Effectiveness (CATIE) Alzheimer trial (Schneider et al., 2006), which compared olanzapine, quetiapine, and risperidone for behavioral problems in patients with Alzheimer's disease, antipsychotics were ineffective or poorly tolerated, with two thirds discontinued after 12 weeks and more than 80% after 36 weeks. The silver lining in this trial was that those patients who were able to tolerate their antipsychotic seemed to derive some benefit from it. SGAs carry a black-box warning about increased risk of death in geriatric patients who receive them for dementia-related psychosis. The risk for cerebrovascular events, such as a stroke, is increased as well. A risk–benefit assessment might still justify a time-limited antipsychotic trial if the behavior is clinically disruptive and other treatments, including non-pharmacologic interventions, have failed.

ADDITIONAL RESOURCES

Book

Coleman M, Gillberg C. *The schizophrenias: A biological approach to the schizophrenia spectrum disorders.* New York: Springer; 1996.—This is a great book that reviews the literature on secondary schizophrenia and offers extensive lists of common and rare disorders to screen for, stratified by treatability.

6 Psychiatric Differential Diagnosis of Psychosis

> **Essential Concepts**
> - Delusional disorder is a psychotic disorder with the hallmark of nonbizarre delusions in an otherwise unremarkable person.
> - Mood disorders can be accompanied by psychosis, including Schneiderian First-Rank Symptoms. In textbook cases, mood disorders are episodic (i.e., have periods of illness clearly delineated from normal), and psychosis is only present during mood episodes, not in the interepisode period.
> - Catatonia has an extensive differential diagnosis that includes medical causes and mood disorders. Catatonic schizophrenia is but one diagnostic consideration.
> - Schizotypal and schizoid personality disorders are nonpsychotic disorders that share attenuated positive and negative symptoms with schizophrenia, respectively. Dissociative phenomena can be confused with psychosis.

"Sometimes paranoia's just having all the facts."
—*William S. Burroughs, 1914–1997, of the Beat Generation*

Once you have excluded drug-induced psychosis and secondary schizophrenia as the cause for psychotic symptoms in a patient, you can then (and only then) turn your attention to primary psychiatric reasons for the psychosis; Table 6.1 presents a comprehensive list of primary psychiatric disorders that can be accompanied by psychosis. These psychiatric disorders are all diagnosed based on clinical features (cross-sectionally and longitudinally) alone, so to diagnose them you must know what they look like in the clinic—there are no laboratory tests that will help you.

DELUSIONAL DISORDER (PARANOIA)

Delusional disorder, the paranoia of late, is a disorder of midlife, with the hallmark of *nonbizarre* delusion(s) in the absence of

TABLE 6.1. **Psychiatric Differential Diagnosis of Psychosis**

Schizophrenia[a]	Catatonia
Schizophreniform disorder, brief psychotic disorders, (ATPD)[a]	Posttraumatic stress disorder (PTSD), dissociation, trance states
Schizoaffective disorder[a]	Personality disorders
Delusional disorder	Paranoid personality disorder
Bipolar disorder	Schizoid and schizotypal personality disorder
Psychotic depression	Borderline and histrionic personality disorder
Late paraphrenia (late-life psychosis)	Autism
Postpartum psychosis	Other pervasive developmental disorders
Obsessive–compulsive disorder (if severe with no insight)	Asperger's syndrome
	Heller's syndrome
Pfropfschizophrenia (schizophrenia "grafted upon" mental retardation)	Rett syndrome
	Nonpathologic psychotic symptoms in general population
Folie á deux	Malingering

ATPD, acute and transient psychotic disorders
[a]Sometimes referred to as "schizophrenia-spectrum disorders."

other prominent psychotic symptoms; only minimal formal thought disorder or hallucinations are allowed. Patients' personalities are intact: In casual conversation you do not suspect a psychiatric disorder unless you happen to come upon the delusion. You are usually able to fit your patient, based on the content of the delusion, into one of these subtypes: persecutory, grandiose, jealous (Othello syndrome), erotomanic (de Clérambault syndrome), and somatic (e.g., Ekbom's syndrome). Some degree of depressive overlay can be present leading to a mistaken diagnosis of psychotic depression.

The degree of social impairment depends on the nature of the delusion, the degree of encapsulation (to which degree patients function normally outside their delusion), and the degree of systematization (i.e., the extent to which the ramifications of a delusional system are connected to a common theme). Grandiose and persecutory delusions are very impairing once these delusions spread and extend into all spheres of life.

Patients with delusional disorders are notoriously difficult to treat, to the point of being untreatable. This is not due to antipsychotic unresponsiveness (they are an effective first-line treatment) but because patients tend to categorically reject psychiatric treatments, as they do not feel ill. Despite great efforts on your part, "insight" is often not forthcoming, and patients come mainly to convince you that they are right and you are wrong. In less severe cases, cognitive–behavioral therapy might lead to some improvement. Sometimes you can provide symptomatic relief with ancillary treatments, e.g., benzodiazepines or antidepressants.

CLINICAL VIGNETTE

An engineer in his 30s lost his job after repeatedly accusing his co-workers of spreading rumors about his sexual orientation. When he confronted an innocent bystander about a perceived insult, he was arrested. He never actually heard anyone talk about him or insult him, but merely had the impression, deduced from gestures, that people were conspiring against him. He had an excellent response to antipsychotics, with complete resolution of persecutory delusions. However, he never acknowledged the possibility that his experiences might have been the result of a psychiatric illness, and only took antipsychotics under duress as part of court-imposed probation.

The management of patients with delusional disorder is further complicated by the real possibility of violence, particularly in patients who feel persecuted or harassed (which can lead to self-defense or preventive action) or loved (which can lead to stalking). A good risk assessment and risk plan is an important part of treatment.

PSYCHOSIS IN MOOD DISORDERS

Psychotic symptoms (i.e., delusions and hallucinations) can occur in primary mood disorders like unipolar depression or bipolar disorder (manic–depressive illness). Unfortunately, there are no pathognomonic psychotic symptoms that allow you to decide if psychosis is part of a mood disorder or schizophrenia.

▼ KEY POINT

An episodic mood disorder (with psychotic mania and/or psychotic depression) is an important diagnostic consideration in any patient with psychotic symptoms. The presence of psychosis during times of euthymia is incompatible with a mood disorder but suggests a schizophrenia-spectrum disorder.

Psychotic Depression

An episode of psychotic depression can represent unipolar or bipolar depression. Without a previous history of mania or a family history of bipolar disorder, the distinction can be impossible to make on clinical grounds alone, although psychomotor retarded-melancholic and atypical episode features (i.e., increased sleep and appetite and leaden paralysis) are more characteristic of bipolar depression (Mitchell et al., 2001). However, bipolar disorder is a disorder of late adolescence, unipolar depression one of middle adulthood: Age of onset alone allows you to make an educated guess about the right diagnosis. Psychotic (unipolar) depression seems to be a distinct subtype of depression, not merely a particularly severe form of depression. A significant minority of patients with depression, about 20%, are affected. Table 6.2 presents a list of differential diagnoses of psychosis with depression.

The full syndrome of psychotic depression is unmistakable. Some patients show extreme psychomotor retardation; others are agitated, ruminating without reprieve about the mood-congruent delusional themes of guilt, worthlessness, and death. Some patients lament their fate and ask to be put out of their misery. They perceive themselves to be a burden to family and society, and suicide can be a constant thought. Paranoid ideation and ideas or delusions of reference are common. Many family members are exasperated at accusations of stealing from the depressed person and the person's delusion of impoverishment. In the extreme of nihilistic delusions, patients deny any future or their own existence, to the point of claiming to be already dead: "Feel me, I am cold" (known as Cotard's syndrome; see Table 1.1).

TABLE 6.2. Differential Diagnose of Psychosis with Depression

Psychotic unipolar depression	Delusional disorder with depressive overlay
Bipolar depression	Dementia with psychosis
Schizophrenia-spectrum disorders	Organic syndromes with psychosis and depression
Postpsychotic depression	

TIP

Consider psychotic depression in all depressed patients refractory to your usual treatment. Psychosis can be subtle, e.g., somatic preoccupation or self-reproach. In some patients paranoia is so prominent that the depressive episode is missed.

If acute suicidality or florid psychosis is present, or if the patient becomes medically compromised (e.g., not eating), a hospitalization will be necessary. An antidepressant combined with an antipsychotic is usually the treatment of choice, followed by electroconvulsive therapy (ECT) if medications fail. Although perphenazine is the most studied antipsychotic for this indication, serotonin reuptake antipsychotics are now first-line agents. Note that full doses of antipsychotics have to be used. Similarly, tricyclic antidepressants have been studied longer, but selective serotonin-reuptake inhibitors (SSRIs) and serotonin–norepinephrine reuptake inhibitors (SNRIs; venlafaxine or duloxetine) are preferred initially. Some patients respond to an antidepressant or antipsychotic alone, but you are not going to know which patients.

For bipolar depression, antidepressants are often added if first-line antidepressant mood stabilizers alone (i.e., lamotrigine and lithium) are not effective. This is controversial as antidepressants are thought to potentially destabilize (i.e., worsen) the long-term course of patients with bipolar disorder (Ghaemi et al., 2003).

Psychotic Mania

Mania is often, but not obligatorily, accompanied by psychosis. In a large sample of 1000 acutely manic patients, 50% were psychotic (Azorin et al., 2007). The typical psychotic symptoms in mania are mood-congruent: Patients are elated, full of energy and plans, and they feel they can take on the world or solve the world's problems. However, Schneiderian symptoms are common as well, and do not argue against a diagnosis of bipolar disorder (Peralta and Cuesta, 1999). Although the mood in mania is classically euphoric, this can quickly change to irritability or frank hostility, particularly if the patient feels you are stymieing his or her plans. A patient whose mood episode is more dysphoric often shows significant paranoia or other psychotic symptoms, leading to a mistaken diagnosis of schizophrenia.

Mania is usually a severe enough illness to require hospitalization (see also Bell's mania in Table 1.1), if only to prevent impulsive and regrettable decisions. Agitation needs to be controlled, and treatment with a mood stabilizer, often with an antipsychotic and/or benzodiazepines, initiated. Following resolution of mania, maintenance treatment with at least one first-line mood stabilizer is necessary.

FOLIE A DEUX

Folie á deux ("infectious insanity," shared psychotic disorder in DSM-IV, induced delusional disorder in ICD-10 terminology) is a psychiatric curiosity that you might never see in your career: In a close relationship, usually in the same family, one person is psychiatrically ill with delusions, and another person adopts the delusional beliefs. Treatment involves separation, with psychiatric treatment for the primarily delusional person (the "primary" or "inducer" or "dominant") and spontaneous recovery of the person in whom delusions were induced (the "secondary" or "acceptor" or "submissive"). There are variants of this involving more than two people. Similar psychologic mechanisms are at play in mass hysteria or cults.

CATATONIA

Catatonic symptoms (see Table 1.4) cut across nosologic boundaries. I follow Taylor and Fink's (2003) suggestion to view catatonia as a syndrome with different etiologies (Table 6.3). In their scheme, catatonic schizophrenia would be seen as (usually) nonmalignant catatonia secondary to a psychotic disorder (i.e., schizophrenia), neuroleptic malignant syndrome (NMS) as a drug-induced form of malignant catatonia. Their approach assigns appropriate importance to catatonic symptoms (which have a very effective and specific treatment in the form of benzodiazepines and ECT) and emphasizes the need for a differential diagnosis that guides your treatment of the underlying etiology. It guards against the inappropriate and outdated assumption that catatonia indicates schizophrenia. Suspect the catatonic syndrome if you see the cardinal signs of immobility, mutism, or stupor accompanied by catalepsy, automatic obedience, or posturing, or (in the absence of cardinal signs) a combination of several catatonic symptoms (criteria proposed by Taylor and Fink).

TABLE 6.3. Classification of Catatonia

Subtypes Based on Severity/Lethality

Nonmalignant catatonia (Kahlbaum's syndrome)	Responds to lorazepam (6–20 mg/day)
Delirious catatonia	Requires high-dose lorazepam or ECT
Malignant catatonia	Requires life support in addition

Specifiers to Indicate Etiology

Secondary to a mood disorder	Secondary to a neurologic disorder
Secondary to a general medical condition or toxic state	Secondary to a psychotic disorder

A psychiatric syndrome with catatonia, periodic catatonia, is a rare familial disorder described in the European literature in which patients have repeated episodes of catatonic stupor or excitement. Between episodes, patients often have residual affective symptoms or show signs of thought disorder or psychosis.

PERSONALITY DISORDERS

In some families you find individuals with clinically diagnosed schizophrenia, as well as "normal" relatives who share some characteristics with their ill relative, albeit at a lesser degree, suggesting some common genetic liability toward schizophrenia. Patients with so-called schizotypal traits show what seem like attenuated positive symptoms: ideas of reference, odd and magical thinking, unusual perceptions, or speech oddities. Interpersonal deficits are usually present in addition to the muffled positive symptoms. When you encounter schizotypal features, consider three possibilities: they can be normal (fairly common as transient, stress-related phenomena during adolescence), they can indicate liability toward schizophrenia, or they can represent prodromal signs of schizophrenia (Bedwell and Donnelly, 2005).

CLINICAL VIGNETTE

I once evaluated a patient who worked as a psychic in the family-owned business of several generations. He communicated with the dead, and he described himself as an "empathic medium," able to "feel" people via their energy fields. He did not have the experiences of thought control, thought insertion, or thought broadcasting. In the right setting with a client, but not usually spontaneously, he heard voices. He was somewhat uncomfortable in social settings because he felt scrutinized and he worried about making a fool of himself. Nevertheless, in the interview he was witty and delightful. He obviously was not impaired vocationally, with the family business going well. Himself a college graduate, he had a brother with schizophrenia.

Think of schizotypal traits (or schizotypal personality disorder, if severe) when you hear about psychic abilities, extrasensory perception (ESP), astrology, or area 51 in New Mexico where "The Government" keeps aliens hidden away. This case illustrates the lack of societal impairment, despite attenuated psychotic symptoms, and the familial aspect of this condition.

By contrast, schizoid traits resemble negative symptoms of schizophrenia. Solitude is preferred to company; consequently, such people are (incorrectly) labeled "antisocial" by the lay public. Often, the only human contact they have is with other family members. They simply do not care about leaving an impression on you; accordingly, the interview is difficult.

Patients with paranoid personality disorder are pathologically suspicious, easily questioning your loyalty, fearing exploitation, always looking for who is going to take advantage of them. Litigation is a real risk, and patients go to great extremes to seek what they think is justice. The border to delusional disorder is not always easy to see.

Sometimes patients with borderline personality disorder have episodes of "micropsychosis," like paranoid ideation or brief hallucinations. Rarely are those experiences sustained. The quality of these psychotic experiences is often different as well (and hence they are probably better regarded as nonpsychotic phenomena). For example, histrionic or borderline patients who endorse hallucinations typically locate voices inside the head, not in external space; they are generally able to acknowledge that the voices are the product of their own mind (not imposed from the outside).

In traumatized patients, consider dissociation (e.g., depersonalization) or trance states. I suspect that some cases of culture-bound, stress-induced psychotic states fall into this category of "psychogenic psychosis."

AUTISM

Even though autism is not characterized by psychosis, social incompetence and concreteness can lead to diagnostic confusion. Some patients with variants of autism (Asperger's syndrome) are misdiagnosed because oddness is taken as signifying psychosis.

There are, of course, obvious similarities between patients with autism and with schizophrenia, leading Eugen Bleuler to identify autism—used descriptively as a deficit in relatedness and partaking in the world, not in the syndromal sense—as a core symptom of schizophrenia (one of his "4 As"). I learned after September 11 that autism is a characteristic of schizophrenia. While most of us were absorbed with the magnitude of the destruction on that day and the implications for our collective future, only one of my patients with schizophrenia made reference to the event in the weeks following the attack; for all other patients it was business as usual, with petty complaints and preoccupation with their own lives.

ADDITIONAL RESOURCES

Books

Ghaemi SN. *Mood disorders: A practical guide.* Philadelphia, PA: Lippincott Williams & Wilkins; 2003.—The corresponding book on mood disorders in this series
Munro A. *Delusional disorder: Paranoia and related illnesses.* Cambridge, UK: Cambridge University Press; 1999.—The standard single-author text on delusional disorder.

Schizophrenia-Spectrum Disorders

Essential Concepts

- Schizophrenia-spectrum disorders are characterized by prominent psychotic symptoms not explained by medical illness or drugs.
- Schizophrenia is a clinical diagnosis based on a combination of characteristic symptoms of sufficient duration and severity (in the absence of other factors that would account for them) that typically begin in late adolescence or early adulthood.
- An unspecific prodromal phase of several years precedes the onset of psychosis. Poor concentration, depression, social withdrawal, and role failure characterize the prodrome.
- Even if a first episode of schizophrenia is successfully treated, there is a high risk of recurrence of psychotic symptoms.
- We are not very good at predicting the eventual outcome of schizophrenia-spectrum disorders, with outcomes ranging from full recovery to severe, unremitting illness requiring institutionalization.

> "It's tough to make predictions,
> especially about the future."
> *Yogi Berra, baseball Hall of Famer, 1972*

The father of psychiatric nosology, Emil Kraepelin, divided severe psychiatric disorders into the episodic mood disorders (i.e., manic–depressive illness or bipolar disorder) and nonepisodic psychotic disorders (i.e., dementia praecox or schizophrenia). Now, 100 years later, we still use this fundamental dichotomy. In his scheme, schizophrenia is the prototypical psychotic illness marked by prominent psychosis in the absence of psychiatric or medical disorders that would explain psychosis; patients who have this disease suffer from some degree of social impairment. In the real world of clinical cases, patients do not always fit the syndrome of schizophrenia: Some patients experience short periods of illness without obvious impairment; others display rather significant admixtures of mood symptoms. To include cases on the edges of narrowly defined schizophrenia, the term "schizophrenia-spectrum conditions" is sometimes used, although disagreement on what conditions to include persists (e.g., some would include schizotypal personality disorder, others delusional disorder) (see Table 6.1 for the use in this book). Yet another term, "nonaffective psychoses" similarly refers to a spectrum of psychotic disorders that includes all psychotic disorders except those in which psychosis is part of a primary mood disorder.

In this chapter I provide a clinical description of the syndrome of schizophrenia that focuses on its natural history. How to make a clinical diagnosis of schizophrenia using current diagnostic criteria is presented in the next chapter.

SCHIZOPHRENIA

The natural history of schizophrenia can be divided into several phases. A stable and clinically asymptomatic premorbid phase gives way to a prodromal period with progressive yet unspecific symptoms until frank psychosis develops. About 50% of patients will become ill between ages 15 and 25, and about 80% between ages 15 and 35. Gender differences exist: More males than females are affected, and females have a later onset (by about 3 to 4 years) and a less virulent disease.

Schizophrenia Prodrome

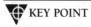 KEY POINT

A prodromal period of 2 to 4 years with unspecific symptoms is often present before acute psychosis suggests the development of schizophrenia. Logically, a prodrome can only be determined retrospectively. About 20% of patients experience no prodrome but have a rather abrupt onset of psychosis.

In medicine, many illnesses are preceded by an unspecific prodromal state during which no diagnosis can be made (e.g., erythema infectiosum or fifth disease, roseola infantum) until certain diagnostic symptoms (telltale rash) appear. Similarly, the full syndrome of schizophrenia with frank psychosis is preceded in most cases by a prodrome that varies in length from several weeks to years. The prodrome can be divided into two phases: a prepsychotic phase and a phase of low-grade, attenuated psychosis that marks the transition to full-blown psychosis. The prepsychotic phase is marked by varied and unspecific symptoms that often result in a psychiatric evaluation and some treatment, usually for depression (Table 7.1). Not only are prodromal symptoms unspecific, but they are also prevalent in normal populations. In one survey of 657 normal 16-year-old high school students, individual prodromal symptoms were endorsed at rates reaching 50% (McGorry et al., 1995).

This prodromal phase of schizophrenia has received much attention, as there is hope that treatment during the prodrome might prevent schizophrenia or ameliorate its effects if treated earlier. The most problematic aspect of treatment during a presumed prodrome is the treatment of patients who will never go on to develop schizophrenia. From prospective studies, we know that only about half of high-risk, presumably prodromal patients will actually develop the full syndrome of schizophrenia. One double-blind trial has shown that olanzapine 5 to 15 mg per day for 1 year given to patients presumed to be prodromal cuts the conversion rate to schizophrenia by half (McGlashan et al., 2006). It is currently unclear what to do beyond 1 year, as it is not clear if the treatment with olanzapine prevents schizophrenia or simply delays the full syndrome.

At this point, close clinical follow-up with symptomatic treatment (e.g., antidepressant for depression) in patients who have a genetic risk for schizophrenia and who develop a decline in function (but no psychosis) is the recommended

TABLE 7.1. Common Prodromal Symptoms of Schizophrenia

Difficulties with concentration
Decreased motivation
Depression
Anxiety and irritability
Difficulties sleeping
Role failure
Social withdrawal

approach. To intervene at the earliest sign of psychosis, long-term follow-up is very important for patients at high risk for schizophrenia.

First Episode of Psychosis

Once a psychosis threshold, defined in terms of both psychotic symptom severity and duration, is crossed, patients are no longer in the prodromal phase of the illness. Rather, they are experiencing their first episode of psychosis. The dividing line between attenuated and frank psychosis is admittedly drawn arbitrarily and not always clear clinically, particularly in the case of a patient with brief, stuttering episodes of low-level psychotic symptoms. Few patients receive treatment for psychosis immediately. The median duration of untreated psychosis (DUP), as the delay in initiation of treatment is called, ranges from 4 to 50 weeks (Marshall et al., 2005). A small group of patients with insidious illness onset receives treatment only after an impressive delay of several years, during which they are quietly psychotic. Diagnostic uncertainty is common during this phase of the illness if mood symptoms and drug use obfuscate the picture.

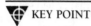 KEY POINT

Depressive symptoms during a first episode of psychosis are the norm, not the exception, in schizophrenia. Up to 75% of patients will have significant depressive symptoms, with 22% meeting severity criteria for full syndromal depression (Koreen et al., 1993).

Multiepisode Patients

After recovery from the initial psychotic episode, almost all patients will experience more episodes. The first few years can be rather "virulent," and frequent hospitalizations and poorly controlled symptoms often interfere with rehabilitation efforts and usually result in a lower "baseline" than where the patient was prior to the onset of schizophrenia (Lieberman et al., 2001). Eventually patients settle at their own level of disability without further decline in function. Cognitive and negative symptoms are the greatest impediment to good function. These two symptom clusters seem to correspond more to a biologic set point for a given patient than being in a reflection of our current treatments.

As patients with schizophrenia grow older, the illness can lessen in its acuity and patients may improve or even recover. However, I have seen geriatric patients worsen simply from decades of not taking care of the brain (e.g., alcoholism, smoking, no exercise).

CLINICAL VIGNETTE

A young college student was hospitalized with florid psychosis following 6 months of depressive symptoms and difficulties concentrating. Because he had used stimulants to concentrate and taken a hallucinogen at a party, a drug-induced psychosis was diagnosed. As a result of the severity of psychosis, antipsychotics were given, and he recovered completely within 2 weeks. Then, 6 months later, the patient was rehospitalized with psychosis, this time without drug use, about 1 month after stopping his antipsychotic.

This is a typical history in that the first psychotic episode, while suggestive of schizophrenia (typical prodromal period), left some diagnostic uncertainty (i.e., the role of drug use). The second episode of psychosis confirmed that he had schizophrenia.

Childhood-Onset Schizophrenia

Childhood-onset schizophrenia (COS), arbitrarily (and inconsistently) defined as onset before age 13, is very rare but not impossible. It is extremely rare before age 10. The prognosis is ominous. Many children have problems that are apparent long before the onset of psychosis: Premorbid function is poor, and children are developmentally delayed in language, motor development, and social skills. The younger a child, the more difficult the diagnosis; normal development (e.g., imaginary friends) must be taken into account to avoid over-diagnosing schizophrenia in childhood. The more persistent the symptoms, the more one should worry about the possibility; the more fleeting or unclear the psychotic symptoms, the more one should consider other diagnoses, e.g., dissociative disorders or autism-spectrum disorders. Family history can help, as genetic loading is more common in COS.

One important developmental task of childhood is schooling; every effort should be made to successfully complete the afflicted child's education.

Late-Onset Schizophrenia

Schizophrenia is generally not considered a disorder of middle or old age, but a significant minority of patients (around 10%) have late-onset schizophrenia (LOS). Dilip Jeste, a researcher specializing in LOS, has argued that age of onset between 40 and 60 years should be considered LOS. Most patients with LOS are female, with better preserved cognition, less promi- nent affective blunting, and no formal thought disorder. The positive-symptom presentation is often paranoid. To me, late-onset paranoid schizophrenia in females with no blunting or thought disorder starts to look very much like delusional disorder.

What if psychosis develops after age 60 or 65? For this age bracket, the term "very late-onset schizophrenia like psy- chosis" has been proposed to indicate the somewhat differ- ent clinical features and probable risk factors. Some authors use the term "late paraphrenia" for cases of late-life psy- chosis: Lonely, never-married, elderly "spinsters" with prob- lems hearing who develop a paranoid psychosis with few other symptoms.

 TIP

I would suggest that you look very hard for medical disorders in any elderly person presenting with psychosis, including early dementia; subclinical delirium; unrecognized, severe alcohol use; or psychotic depression before diagnosing one of the nonaffective psychotic disorders. Make sure patients get eyeglasses and hearing aids.

BRIEF AND INTERMITTENT PSYCHOTIC DISORDERS

Some patients experience brief psychotic episodes with return to good baseline function between episodes and no significant residual impairment. Clinically, the onset tends to be rather acute, and confusion and bewilderment are prominent; patients are described as "perplexed." Those patients with such atypical psychoses present a diagnostic dilemma. Although it is certainly conceivable that they represent a forme fruste of schizophrenia, they might also be very different illnesses (Marneros, 2006). The clinical point here is that narrowly defined schizophrenia assumes a particular disease course, marked by some form of deterioration and often a typical prodrome. Until we better understand the pathophysiology of schizophrenia, we should be conservative in diagnosing it and consider somebody undiagnosed, when faced with atypical psychosis.

In DSM-IV terminology, such atypical patients are classified as having a brief psychotic disorder if symptoms of psychosis last for at least 1 day but for less than 30 days, or schizophreniform disorder if symptoms last for less than 6 months. Acute and transient psychotic disorders (ATPD) and *bouffée délirante* (in French-speaking countries like Haiti) are other terms applied to this patient group. Interestingly, atypical cases of psychosis are more common in non-Western cultures than in the United States or Europe, with many societies having their own term for these acute-onset good-prognosis illnesses. "Psychogenic" psychosis as a form of psychosis induced by severe stress has been proffered as a possible mechanism to explain this phenomenon.

SCHIZOAFFECTIVE DISORDER

Some patients experience the symptoms of schizophrenia and bipolar disorder simultaneously and equally prominently, leading to a diagnosis of schizoaffective disorder. The necessity for this residual diagnostic category is a challenge for nosology and has led to the idea of a "unitary psychosis," in which any patient can be located on a continuum between schizophrenia like illness and bipolar like illness, with varying admixtures of mood and psychotic symptoms.

According to DSM-IV, schizoaffective disorder can be diagnosed if a manic or depressive syndrome has been present concurrent with characteristic psychotic symptoms of schizophrenia, if psychotic symptoms have persisted for at least 2 weeks when there were no prominent mood symptoms, and if mood symptoms were present "for a substantial portion of the active and residual phase." It should be obvious that these complex rules are open to interpretation (and require knowledge of longitudinal symptoms that is often impossible to ascertain). Consequently, some have pointed out that schizoaffective disorder is one of the most unreliable diagnoses (Vollmer-Larsen et al., 2006), which of course raises the question why you should use the term at all.

When I am faced with a patient who seems to be suffering from both syndromes, I try to decide between three clinical possibilities to guide treatment:

- The patient has a severe form of bipolar disorder and not schizophrenia. Some patients with bipolar disorder have episodes of psychosis severe enough to overshadow the mood component. This is important to recognize since every effort, including use of electroconvulsive therapy, should be made to achieve remission from this episode before it becomes chronic, and to prevent future episodes with mood stabilizers. Consider this possibility particularly if there is a strong family history of clear-cut bipolar disorder.

- The patient has schizophrenia and comorbid dysthymia or recurrent depression. Patients with schizophrenia are vulnerable to demoralization or depressive episodes, particularly at times of stress. This conceptualization suggests the need for maintenance treatment with antipsychotics but also gives you very specific ideas about the treatment of the comorbid mood disorders, including nonpharmacologic approaches.

- The patient has "true" schizoaffective disorder. I accept the limitations of making diagnoses based on symptoms alone and occasionally will use this category for those patients who are not better captured by the above categories and in whom psychosis and mood seem to be intertwined and equally prominent. This will often be the case in patients with substance use or in patients who are early in the course of schizophrenia. I consider this a schizophrenia variant, but the diagnosis suggests the long-term need for antipsychotics as well as mood stabilizers and antidepressants.

A special case of mood symptoms in schizophrenia is the patient with schizophrenia who develops postpsychotic depression. This scenario should be clear from the longitudinal history. The depressive episode is treatable with antidepressants. Lastly mood symptoms during exacerbations of psychosis should be treated by optimizing antipsychotics (Levinson et al., 1999).

OUTCOME

"It's tough to make predictions," Yogi Berra is supposed to have said, "especially about the future." The pioneering work of the Swiss psychiatrist Eugen Bleuler of the famous Burghoelzli Clinic in Zürich, Switzerland and his son, Manfred Bleuler, showed that there is no one course or outcome of schizophrenia. A useful analogy is multiple sclerosis, which allows for episodic cases with no disability, episodic cases with accrued disability over time, or a progressive subtype (Lublin and Reingold, 1996). As a rule of thumb, the outcome of schizophrenia can be depicted in four quadrants:

1. 25% have one or few psychotic episodes, usually of acute onset, from which they completely recover. These "good-prognosis cases" seem to be more common in the developing world. In the United States, this quadrant might be much smaller, more like 10%.
2. 25% have episodes with good symptomatic recovery but some degree of functional limitation; patients are able to live independently.
3. 25% have episodes with incomplete recovery and hence significant interepisode residual symptoms. This group of patients needs substantial support from family or the state.
4. 25% have a very poor prognosis, with relentless, impairing symptoms requiring continued hospitalization or institutionalization (Kraepelinian subtype of schizophrenia).

ADDITIONAL RESOURCES

Web Site

http://www.schizophrenia.com/earlypsychosis.htm—A list of links to all first-episode programs by country and state.

Book

Yung A, Phillips L, McGorry PD. *Treating schizophrenia in the prodromal phase.* London: Taylor & Francis; 2004.—From the Australian pioneers in prodromal schizophrenia.

8 Diagnosing Schizophrenia— Clinical Approach

> **Essential Concepts**
> - Schizophrenia is a clinical diagnosis you can make if typical symptoms are present long enough and are severe enough in the absence of other causative factors (i.e., drug use, medical illness, or other psychiatric disorders).
> - Schizophrenia can be reliably diagnosed using criteria-based diagnostic schemes (e.g., DSM-IV or ICD-10).
> - Typical symptoms of schizophrenia are psychosis and negative symptoms, but other symptom domains (cognition, affect, catatonia) need to be assessed as well. Use a rating scale to track symptom severity over time.
> - Psychosis by longitudinal symptom review is key for a diagnosis of schizophrenia, but not if the patient is psychotic in your office.

Madness is tonic and invigorating. It makes the sane more sane. The only ones who are unable to profit by it are the insane."
Henry Miller, American writer, 1891–1980

The syndrome of schizophrenia, as described in the previous chapter, can be reliably diagnosed using well-established criteria such as those developed by the American Psychiatric Association or the World Health Organization (Table 8.1). These diagnostic criteria represent a consensus among experts and identify narrowly defined, core schizophrenia.

Your diagnosis of the schizophrenia syndrome is made *clinically*; the name (or label) that you give your patient's disease is based on criteria for classification (of which there are competing schemes). Yet the clinical phenomena are much richer than the diagnostic criteria, so avoid resorting to

TABLE 8.1. Key Diagnostic Features of Schizophrenia (according to DSM-IV[a])

Active-phase symptoms

One characteristic symptom from this list:
  Typical hallucinations (i.e., running commentary, conversing voices)
  Bizarre delusions

or

Two symptoms from this list:
  Delusions
  Hallucinations
  Disorganized speech
  Disorganized behavior or catatonia
  Negative symptoms

Duration of symptoms

6 months of illness (*including prodrome*); 1 month of acute symptoms

Functional decline

Required

---

[a] This list is based on the fourth edition of the American Psychiatric Association's *Diagnostic and Statistical Manual*, DSM-IV. Other diagnostic schemes differ in the criteria required for a diagnosis of schizophrenia. For example, the World Health Organization's 10th edition of the *International Classification of Diseases*, ICD-10, requires only 1 month of acute symptoms and no functional decline.

"checklist psychiatry" in which all you know about the disease is a limited list of symptoms that you check off your clipboard (Freudenreich et al., 2004).

DIAGNOSING SCHIZOPHRENIA FOR THE FIRST TIME

All psychiatric disorders are diagnosed by typical symptoms and a typical course *only after "organic" causes have been ruled out.* I do not like to call schizophrenia a "diagnosis of exclusion," as this often implies "by default"; schizophrenia is still diagnosed positively, only if typical signs and symptoms and a typical course are present.

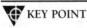 **KEY POINT**

Psychosis does not equal schizophrenia: There are many etiologies of psychosis, with schizophrenia merely one diagnostic possibility. A differential diagnosis to exclude other reasons for psychosis is necessary.

To diagnose schizophrenia, answer the following questions, not necessarily in this order:

- How did psychiatric symptoms develop over time and what symptoms are currently present (see Chapter 2)?
- Is a delirium present (see Chapter 3)?
- Could this be a drug-induced psychosis (see Chapter 4)?
- Is one of the secondary schizophrenias responsible for the psychosis (see Chapter 5)?
- Are the clinical features more typical for other psychiatric disorders, particularly bipolar disorder or psychotic depression (see Chapter 6)?
- Does your clinical diagnosis of schizophrenia fulfill the diagnostic criteria for schizophrenia as described above? It usually will; however, atypical cases will not fit.

Patients with schizophrenia can have different combinations of symptoms, and no two patients will look alike. Depending on the exact admixture of symptoms, different historical subtypes (or types) have been described—i.e., catatonic, disorganized (hebephrenic), paranoid, undifferentiated, or residual. The subtypes are neither stable over time nor very useful, in part because most patients fall into the undifferentiated or residual category. Instead of subtyping patients, I describe their symptom cluster profile, that is, which of the following symptom cluster(s) dominate(s) in a given patient: positive symptoms (separated into disorganization and delusions/hallucinations), negative symptoms, cognitive symptoms, or affective symptoms (includes excitability, dysphoria, suicidality); rarely, a motor symptom cluster (with catatonia) is clinically discernible. Measure cross-sectional symptom severity with a rating scale—for example, the Brief Psychiatric Rating Scale (BPRS) and the Global Assessment of Functioning (GAF) (see Appendix B).

CONFIRMING SCHIZOPHRENIA IN THE ESTABLISHED PATIENT

You will often take over the care of established patients who come to you on maintenance antipsychotics with a "history of chronic schizophrenia." The basics of confirming a diagnosis of schizophrenia are not different from diagnosing new patients, except that you do not have to reinvent the wheel: Use data already collected for you.

TIP

Get collateral information that is both recent and distant. From patients with a long history of schizophrenia, get the first and last hospital discharge summaries to learn how it all started, as well as to get a recent view and a chronologic summary, if you are lucky. Be aware that diagnostic standards and treatments have changed. In the United States, 1980 is a watershed year because of the introduction of a narrow concept of (DSM-III) schizophrenia, also known as the neo-Kraepelinian approach.

In some patients you will be able to make a diagnosis of schizophrenia simply because of the patient's presentation with typical symptoms despite treatment (if you assume that the patient's symptoms are stable). However, some treated patients are fairly asymptomatic (the medicine is working). This can leave you with the dilemma of not having seen florid psychopathology yourself and having to make diagnostic and treatment decisions based on second-hand information. In diagnosing these patients, do not dismiss schizophrenia because:

- "He is doing too well for schizophrenia." This stems from the perception that all patients with schizophrenia must have a chronic, debilitating illness. This assumption is simply untrue.
- The patient is not psychotic when interviewed. I am treating many patients whom I have never seen psychotic because they have stayed on maintenance antipsychotics and never had a relapse.
- The patient seems to be a good "historian" (a useful, albeit obviously incorrect, term unless that patient has a university degree in history) and convinces you that previous treaters were incorrect about the diagnosis. Lack of insight into symptoms and poor memory can distort the truth.

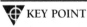 KEY POINT

Most of the time, most patients with treated schizophrenia are not psychotic.

COMMON DIAGNOSTIC MISTAKES

Psychiatric diagnoses are based on cross-sectional and longi-*tudinal* symptom review. I think most mistakes are made when a diagnosis is based on acute presentations only. Admittedly, unless you live with your patients in a state hospital (like the alienists used to), you will, in fact, have only a rather incomplete knowledge about longitudinal symptoms. What is more, patients are almost never untreated; therefore, you see fully or partially treated syndromes. Nevertheless, strive to avoid these mistakes:

- Schizophrenia is not diagnosed because of prominent mood symptoms during an exacerbation of schizophrenia, even though mood symptoms are not prominent during the longitudinal course of the illness.
- Schizophrenia is missed because symptoms are falsely attributed to drug use. Conversely, schizophrenia is diagnosed even though substance use alone can explain the presentation.
- Schizophrenia is diagnosed because dissociative symptoms and transient psychotic experiences (e.g., mild paranoid ideation or stress-induced hallucinations) are misinterpreted as evidence for schizophrenia.
- "Cultural" explanations are proffered to falsely reject schizophrenia or to inappropriately invoke schizophrenia. In people from other cultures or with other religions, you are occasionally unable to judge if psychosis is present: Ask somebody from within the culture in order to avoid misdiagnosis. However, the syndrome of schizophrenia is usually easily recognizable, regardless of where the patient is from, and the "cultural" aspect a mere distraction. Nevertheless, "pathoplastic" (illness-shaping) influences of culture on diseases and their symptoms can lead to lack of congruity with DSM categories (e.g., *bouffée délirante* of Haiti: an acute, confusional psychotic disorder that resolves quickly—one example of a "culture-bound" syndrome).
- The patient is diagnosed with schizophrenia because the patient looks psychiatrically ill even though criteria are not met. Consider variants of autism.

Let me add one last diagnostic mistake: Schizophrenia is diagnosed because of psychosis for which no cause can be found, even though the person is otherwise well. Psychotic symptoms without clinical significance were surprisingly common in a community survey in the Netherlands (The Netherlands Mental Health Survey and Incidence Study, or NEMESIS), in which almost 2 out of 10 people endorsed some form of psychotic symptom, an observation consistent with a psychosis continuum concept (which is the idea expressed in the epigraph to this chapter, a quote from Henry Miller) (Verdoux and van Os, 2002).

COMMON DIAGNOSTIC OMISSIONS

Your goal at the end of the interview is not only to establish a diagnosis of schizophrenia and to characterize the severity of the psychiatric symptom clusters, but also to clearly rule in or rule out other psychiatric diagnoses.

 KEY POINT

Don't just stop once you have diagnosed schizophrenia, but consider other, additional diagnoses that can complicate treatment or are amenable to treatment. Schizophrenia can be overbearing, often seeming to tower above other problems. However, once psychosis is controlled, it is the "minor" diagnoses and the patient's cognitive style (to use David Shapiro's term) that matter most in treatment!

Specifically, consider the following psychiatric diagnostic questions:

- Is a personality disorder present? Cognitive styles matter; in particular, recognize antisocial or borderline traits, which greatly complicate your clinical management.
- Is cognitive impairment so severe that dementia could be diagnosed?
- Are other syndromal diagnoses present? Consider recurrent depression, posttraumatic stress disorder, panic disorder, social phobia, and obsessive–compulsive disorder (OCD). It remains to be seen if "schizo-obsessive disorder" is a valid subtype of co-occurring OCD plus schizophrenia.

ADDITIONAL RESOURCES
Books

Two comprehensive, competing textbooks of schizophrenia you can choose from:

Hirsch SR, Weinberger DR, eds. *Schizophrenia*. 2nd ed. Malden, MA: Blackwell; 2003.

Lieberman JA, Stroup TS, Perkins DO, eds. *The American Psychiatric Publishing textbook of schizophrenia*. Washington, DC: American Psychiatric Publishing; 2006.

Article

Jansson LB, Parnas J. Competing definitions of schizophrenia: What can be learned from polydiagnostic studies? *Schizophr Bull*. 2006;[Epub ahead of print]—Read this article to understand the vexing problem of validity of psychiatric diagnosis (and the limitations of our current approach to diagnosing schizophrenia).

III

TREATMENT OF PSYCHOTIC DISORDERS

9 Emergency Management of Acute Psychosis

> **Essential Concepts**
> - During all steps of the emergency evaluation of a psychotic patient, ensure the safety of the patient, staff, and other patients in the emergency department (ED).
> - Agitation is a behavioral emergency that needs to be treated aggressively. Recognize the symptoms of agitation and offer medications early. However, the ultimate goal of the emergency evaluation is diagnosis, so avoid oversedation.
> - The most important determination in the ED will be if a psychotic patient is medically ill or delirious, intoxicated or withdrawing, or if the patient suffers from a primary psychiatric illness. The three are not mutually exclusive.
> - Do not discharge a patient with psychosis from the ED unless you are confident about your diagnosis and the feasibility of your follow-up plan.

> "Coolness and absence of heat and haste indicate fine qualities."
> —*Ralph Waldo Emerson, American transcendentalist, 1803–1882*

In the emergency setting, you might have to treat psychotic patients before you have a firm (or any) diagnosis. Consider diagnosis to be a reiterative process, and the process outlined below is not necessarily sequential. At all times, remember Emerson's quote and approach psychotic patients calmly and without haste.

INITIAL STABILIZATION FOR SAFETY

First, you need to decide where in the ED acutely psychotic patients need to go: Can they simply wait in the general waiting area with a family member until they can be seen, should they be secured in a locked room, do they need to be restrained, or do they need to go to the medical side (if the psychiatric ED is separate from the medical ED)?

Symptoms of psychosis are often very disturbing to patients and may lead to poor judgments regarding safe behavior. Agitation is a combination of physical signs involving aimless movements that suggest internal emotional distress. Staring intensely, hand wringing, fidgeting, pacing, clenched fists, shadowboxing, posturing, and pounding on doors or walls are all signs of agitation. Some patients may arrive agitated or combative, whereas others are calm until they recognize that their families have coaxed them into going to the ED under false pretenses. Patients might agree to an evaluation if they perceive that you are at least considering "letting them go" after the evaluation. Never promise that you will let a patient go if the patient talks with you, but inform the patient that talking with you is a *sine qua non* for possible release.

 TIP

A psychotic patient in the ED should be viewed as potentially violent until proven otherwise. To gauge potential for violence, review all accompanying materials before you go to see the patient.

A series of treatments can be offered to decrease a patient's distress. Offers of food and drink, warm blankets, a trip to the restroom, or a more comfortable place to wait may decrease anxiety and help you to form an alliance. Acknowledge the patient's power to make decisions and provide information about the ED process in a calm voice. Clear limit-setting about safe behaviors in the ED also sets the stage for offers of medication if the patient is unable to behave in a safe manner. If a patient appears agitated, keep yourself safe by maintaining at least an arm's distance from the patient, meet in a location where you can leave the room quickly, and limit the items in the room that could be picked up or thrown.

If a patient requires medication, follow the principles below for acute treatment with medications (see next paragraph and EM Card Acute Behavioral Disturbance in Appendix A for some commonly used regimens). If done correctly, medications are a safe way to protect patients, caregivers, and other patients from injury. Appropriate use of medication also reduces the time that a patient might spend in physical restraints. Physical restraint, a last resort in the management of acute agitation, can be necessary and lifesaving for extremely agitated patients.

Whenever possible, use oral medications in cooperative patients. A show of force might convince patients to cooperate and not risk a fight. Experts disagree if benzodiazepines alone are as effective for agitation as antipsychotics with or without a benzodiazepine. Several second-generation antipsychotics are now available in intramuscular (IM) preparations (i.e., aripiprazole, olanzapine, and ziprasidone). I am more likely to use second-generation antipsychotics in the ED setting if schizophrenia is the reason for agitation (consistent with Lukens et al., 2006). Otherwise, I use the haloperidol–lorazepam combination, which has an excellent track record regarding both safety and efficacy for any acute behavioral emergency. In some situations, it is probably safer to use benzodiazepines alone—e.g., antipsychotics increase risk for neuroleptic malignant syndrome (NMS) in patients with amphetamine intoxication. Make sure not to use antipsychotics if catatonia or NMS is a possibility. Also, do not use "rapid neuroleptization" (i.e., the use of large loading doses of antipsychotics), as this strategy does not confer any benefit. Note that agitated patients in alcohol or benzodiazepine withdrawal might need substantially higher doses of benzodiazepines than commonly recommended for acute agitation from other causes.

The following are common mistakes that I have seen in the use of medications for acute agitation:

- An initial dose is given but not repeated in a timely fashion, even though the patient is not calm. Agitation is a behavioral emergency and must be treated like any medical emergency: With close follow-up *until the emergency situation is resolved.*
- Patients are given too much medication and are put to sleep. Your goal is to examine the patient to arrive at a diagnosis that will guide treatment, not to have a patient sleep in the ED.
- The standard cocktail (of haloperidol plus lorazepam plus benztropine) is repeated until the patient has developed anticholinergic toxicity and/or akathisia.

INITIAL DIAGNOSIS AND DIFFERENTIAL DIAGNOSIS

Once the patient is calm, perform a physical examination, a mental status examination, and order some initial labs. A delirium is a medical emergency and always has a medical cause that needs to be identified and treated, if possible (see Chapter 3 on delirium workup and treatment). In textbook cases, a delirious patient is inattentive and has obvious memory problems, whereas a psychiatrically psychotic patient has no problems in those realms. In reality, I have examined many psychotic patients who have great difficulties relating their history coherently or who do not cooperate sufficiently with my examination. Sometimes sedating medications were given, which obfuscated the picture further. You will have to rely on your overall impression and serial examinations. Severe mania can appear delirious, hence the term "delirious mania."

There is no generally agreed-upon "medical clearance" that every psychotic patient must have in the ED, but I think it is reasonable to obtain routine labs to exclude intoxication, withdrawal, or common, treatable medical illnesses as the cause for psychosis, supplemented by lumbar puncture, electroencephalogram (EEG), and computed tomography/magnetic resonance imaging (CT/MRI), if indicated clinically (use Table 3.3 as a guide for what to include in your workup). History with initial presentation, vital signs, your examination, and initial labs should allow you to triage patients who are referred to the ED for "acute psychosis" into one of these subgroups:

Young, combative patient, possibly psychotic. Any combative patient should be considered potentially psychotic (and vice versa). Other common diagnoses in the differential include intoxication (e.g., PCP), withdrawal from a substance (e.g., alcohol), delirium, or a personality disorder. History and a urine drug screen (UDS) might help. Note, however, that the UDS does not screen for all drugs of abuse (e.g., LSD, ketamine). Paranoid patients can be violent, particularly if drug use is involved. Irritable mania can also lead to a very volatile presentation.

Older patient with recent onset of psychosis. Until proven otherwise, any patient without a psychiatric history who presents with psychosis after the age of 40 should be considered medically ill, most likely delirious. The older the patient, the less likely this will be an initial presentation of one of the psychotic disorders. Elderly, delirious patients can be quietly psychotic and withdrawn. Always perform a urinalysis for these patients, because a urinary tract infection is the most common cause of mental status change in older patients. Other diagnoses to consider are dementia with psychosis and psychotic depression or psychotic mania.

Young patient with first episode of psychosis: "first-episode patient." A typical history will show a college student with a decline in psychosocial function over several months or sometimes even years, who has become acutely psychotic. These patients commonly refer to their psychotic symptoms as "anxiety" when they first present to the ED. Question the specific feelings and experiences associated with the anxiety, and listen for new-onset paranoia. Look for a family history of psychotic illness. Although drug use is often present (particularly cannabis use), it is often incidental, and the psychotic episode does not resolve spontaneously after drug use is stopped.

Patient with longstanding history of psychotic illness (schizophrenia or bipolar disorder): "acute on chronic." For most patients, schizophrenia is a chronic illness with acute exacerbations, even with treatment. Although an acute illness exacerbation is the most likely cause in this scenario, the reason for the exacerbation must be clarified. Important factors can include antipsychotic medication partial adherence or nonadherence, alcohol and drug use, or significant environmental changes (e.g., a new staff member at the group home). Some patients will be marginally compensated to begin with, and any worsening will put them at the hospital level of care. Psychogenic polydipsia is a complication in 10% of patients with chronic schizophrenia who periodically develop dangerously low sodium levels from drinking water. Hyponatremia can cause mental status changes and seizures; ask the group home or families about excessive water intake. An intercurrent medical illness (e.g., pneumonia) must always be considered as a potential cause for worsening of a patient's psychotic symptoms, and a careful review of medical history and examination (e.g., chest X-ray) is necessary. If the patient is homeless, he or she may be at higher risk for new medical illnesses or exacerbation of chronic ones (e.g., skin infections, tuberculosis, diabetes), either from limited access to general medical care or the living conditions on the street or in a shelter. A thorough physical examination should be done, including a skin examination, and one should have a low threshold for any indicated tests and laboratory studies.

"Frequent flyer" with "psychosis." All emergency rooms have a handful of patients that visit the ED frequently. Such patients often have borderline or antisocial personality disorder diagnoses and usually misuse drugs. Psychosis could be present (e.g., from drug use) or malingered (including by patients with schizophrenia who have nowhere to go). You might not be able to clarify this in the ED setting (see Chapter 2 for malingering).

INITIATION OF TREATMENT SPECIFIC FOR DIAGNOSIS

In some EDs, "definite treatment" will be initiated if the diagnosis has become clear during the evaluation. Restarting previously effective antipsychotics in patients with schizophrenia who have become nonadherent is reasonable; note that you might have to give a lower dose, depending on the duration of missed antipsychotics. If psychosis is thought to be drug induced (e.g., cocaine-induced psychosis), consider delaying treatment with an antipsychotic to clarify the diagnosis, unless the patient is exhibiting agitated or dangerous behavior. In some cases (e.g., chronic use of crystal methamphetamine or cocaine), the drug-induced psychosis may continue even after the period of intoxication. In these cases, antipsychotic medications can be helpful. Acutely manic patients will benefit from the sedating effects of benzodiazepines and can also receive a loading dose of valproate (20 to 30 mg/kg/day) almost immediately upon arrival at the ED.

APPROPRIATE DISPOSITION

When can you discharge a patient with psychosis from the ED? The answer to this question has to do more with risk and social factors than with psychiatric diagnosis per se. The correct disposition requires clinical experience and should not be done without consultation with a physician experienced in emergency psychiatry. Consider the following situations as a starting point for your considerations:

- If psychosis from drug use resolves in the ED in the expected time course, discharge and referral to a substance use outpatient program might be reasonable.
- If a chronically psychotic patient seems calm and cooperative in the ED after a behavioral incident in a group home, work with the group home to resolve the issue that got the patient upset; at a minimum, clarify what a brief psychiatric admission is supposed to accomplish.
- Do not overburden family (and patients) with clinical responsibilities; in most cases, a potentially dangerous patient with psychosis should be admitted to the hospital even if the family is willing to take the patient home (with some education, most families will agree with you).
- Psychiatric hospitalizations are not without risks (i.e., stigma). If possible, avoid hospitalization for first-episode patients but initiate treatment in an outpatient setting, *unless this is unsafe or follow-up is unlikely or cannot be arranged in the ED.*
- Hospitalize any psychotic patient who is dangerous or gravely disabled even if the patient does not agree to the

admission (refer to the civil commitment laws in your state regarding involuntary admission).

- You might have to admit a patient who seeks admission and whom you suspect of malingering psychosis. Don't take it personally.
- Think twice before you discharge a psychotic patient who was brought to the ED because of violence, simply because the patient is calm during the evaluation and has a good explanation for everything that happened.
- Think twice before you discharge a manic patient unless mania is just beginning and family members are confident that they can supervise medications. Patients with acute mania have no appreciation of their illness and the need for treatment.

ADDITIONAL RESOURCES

Articles

Marco CA, Vaughan J. Emergency management of agitation in schizophrenia. *Am J Emerg Med.* 2005;23:767–776.—Review that includes discussion of newer antipsychotics.

Lukens TW, Wolf SJ, Edlow JA, et al. Clinical policy: Critical issues in the diagnosis and management of the adult psychiatric patient in the emergency department. *Ann Emerg Med.* 2006;47:79–99.—Recommendations for acute agitation from the American College of Emergency Physicians.

Phase-Specific Treatment of Schizophrenia

> **Essential Concepts**
> - Treatment during the three stages of illness (i.e., acute, stabilization, and stable maintenance phase) tries to achieve symptom response, symptom resolution, and symptom remission and recovery, respectively.
> - Symptomatic remission in schizophrenia is defined as a relative absence of positive and negative symptoms, not a complete freedom from symptoms, for at least 6 months. Functional recovery is only possible for a minority of patients (less than 20%).
> - Antipsychotics are the basis for relapse prevention. Frequent relapse disrupts rehabilitation efforts and hinders sustained remission and eventual recovery.
> - Always focus on rehabilitation and optimal function, even in the presence of symptoms (freedom from symptoms might not be possible).

> "Never, never, never, never give up."
> —*Winston Churchill, English statesman, 1874-1965*

> "However beautiful the strategy, you should occasionally look at the results."
> —*Winston Churchill, English statesman, 1874-1965*

The treatment of schizophrenia can be thought of as proceeding through phases, not necessarily sharply demarcated, with each phase having different treatment goals (Table 10.1).

ACUTE PHASE

Usually, but not always, initial treatment for an acute psychotic episode is provided in the hospital, where antipsychotics are initiated with the expectation of response. Ancillary medications (e.g., benzodiazepine or valproate acid) are often prescribed to reduce the severity of the patient's

**TABLE 10.1. Phase-Specific Treatment Goals
for Schizophrenia**

Acute Phase (Response)	Prevent harm and control psychotic behavior Achieve symptom response, reduce symptom severity Build alliance with patient and family
Stabilization Phase (Resolution)	Achieve resolution of symptoms and early remission Prevent early relapse Early readjustment to community living Monitor and address side effects
Stable (Maintenance) Phase (Remission and Recovery)	Sustained symptom remission Improve function and quality of life Monitor and address demoralization and suicidality Monitor and address long-term iatrogenic morbidity Find meaning in life despite illness

psychopathology. This acute illness phase often provides a window of opportunity for engaging the family.

"Response" merely signifies a reduction in symptoms severity, usually quantified as a percent decrease on a rating scale of psychopathology. While some response (e.g., a 20% reduction in psychopathology) is achieved by the majority of first-episode patients, even such small reductions in symptom severity can take several weeks in some patients (Emsley et al., 2006). Patience is required, and "pushing the dose" of the antipsychotic is unnecessary: You cannot accelerate the resolution of psychosis once dopamine receptors are sufficiently blocked; it takes time for a complex delusional system to resolve. Yet, in multiepisode patients, the greatest reduction in symptoms occurs in the first few weeks of treatment (Agid et al., 2003), and many patients show signs of response almost immediately after treatment is initiated (such as a reduction in excitability). A modern view of antipsychotic response rejects the idea of a delayed response. Instead, it posits an immediate action of antipsychotics with accrued benefits over time (Kapur et al., 2005).

STABILIZATION PHASE

During this illness phase, the main focus remains on symptoms. When patients are discharged, they are still rather symptomatic. However, given time (and assuming an antipsychotic-responsive form of schizophrenia), positive symptoms are expected to remit completely while other problems, particularly side effects, negative symptoms, and depression (postpsychotic depression), become the focus of treatment. For many first-episode patients, this early adjustment period following a psychiatric hospitalization will last anywhere from 3 months to 1 year.

Although many first-episode patients achieve short-term resolution of symptoms initially, the goal of sustained remission is often elusive because patients relapse after prematurely stopping antipsychotics. In fact, fewer than 50% of first-episode patients are still on antipsychotics 1 year after their first episode. The resulting deterioration may represent a failure to achieve sufficient clinical stability, as adherence to antipsychotics is one of the best predictors of good outcome. Partial adherence and intermittent drug use are key factors in relapse.

STABLE PHASE (MAINTENANCE PHASE)

In this phase, you move beyond symptom management to improving function and quality of life, and to prevent the ultimate bad outcome: premature death. Preventing relapse to maintain remission is the *sine qua non* of rehabilitation and recovery. Long-term health issues, such as possible medical morbidity, are becoming more urgent considerations, necessitating a focus on wellness and lifestyle choices (see Chapter 21). Demoralization and suicide can become urgent matters if patients are unable to adjust to a life different from the one envisioned (see Chapter 28).

Remission (Relapse Prevention)

Only recently have remission criteria been developed (Table 10.2). Once sustained remission (for more than 6 months) has been achieved, it becomes important *to keep* patients in remission. This cannot be overemphasized, as the foundation for any further improvement hinges on the ability to participate in treatment and life. For most patients with narrowly defined schizophrenia (e.g., DSM-IV or ICD-10

TABLE 10.2. Consensus Criteria for Symptomatic Remission in Schizophrenia

1) Focus on three core psychopathologic symptom dimensions (delusions and hallucinations; disorganization; negative symptoms)
2) Symptom severity below clinically significant threshold for all core domains (i.e., mild or less)
3) Sustained symptomatic remission for at least 6 months

Remission does not require complete freedom from symptoms
Remission focuses on symptomatic, not functional recovery

Adapted from Andreasen NC, Carpenter Jr. WT, Kane JM, et al. Remission in schizophrenia: proposed criteria and rationale for consensus. *Am J Psychiatry.* 2005;162:441–449.

schizophrenia), this is a chronic remitting and relapsing illness. Pretending that this is untrue is not helpful, and maintenance treatment with an antipsychotic will be required, hence the maintenance phase.

⊕ KEY POINT

The psychotic relapse risk after discontinuing antipsychotics is very high for both first-episode and multiepisode patients. A seminal study of first-episode patients showed a broadly defined relapse rate (re-emergence of symptoms, not necessarily hospitalization) approaching 100% after 2 years (Gitlin et al., 2001). In multiepisode patients, discontinuing maintenance antipsychotics increases the relapse risk fivefold even with maintenance treatment, 30% of patients per year will have a relapse.

Intermittent treatment (treatment with antipsychotics only during acute illness phases) is not as effective, at least not for multiepisode patients, and is discouraged for most patients (Carpenter et al., 1990).

In clinical reality, most patients will want to stop their medications at some point. This is true for both first-episode and multiepisode patients. It is prudent to plan for this since early detection of relapse is possible and a full relapse can be averted (Gitlin et al., 2001). If a decision is made to stop antipsychotics, try to do the following to minimize the risk of a major relapse:

• Taper antipsychotics over many months, if feasible (to reduce withdrawal effects).

- Develop an individualized relapse signature based on the knowledge about how previous episodes developed.
- Involve the family in the decision and develop a crisis plan with them.
- Have a frank discussion about the risks of relapse and the risks and benefits of treatment. In some cases, advise against discontinuation if psychosis was dangerous, and document that discontinuing the antipsychotic is against medical advice.
- If your patient is asking for a treatment-free period, argue for antipsychotic continuation until a major milestone is reached (e.g., finishing college).
- Inform patients that relapse risk is probably stable and does not decrease with time.

 KEY POINT

The goal of maintenance treatment with antipsychotics for schizophrenia is prevention of relapse, not comprehensive treatment of schizophrenia (Carpenter, 2001). For almost all patients with schizophrenia, antipsychotics are merely the foundation for remission without relapse as the basis for recovery.

Recovery (Rehabilitation)

Ultimately, patients need to rebuild their lives. Liberman and Kopelowicz (Liberman et al., 2002), two rehabilitation specialists from the University of California in Los Angeles (UCLA), have proposed specific recovery criteria, including four domains that must be met for at least 2 years: symptom remission (positive as well as negative symptoms); appropriate role function (part-time work or school, homemaker); ability to perform day-to-day living tasks without supervision; and social interactions with people outside the family.

Statistically, the odds for such defined full recovery are not good. In one trial of first-episode patients, only 14% met the above UCLA recovery criteria 5 years later (Robinson et al., 2004). For some patients, freedom from symptoms and independence in a complex society are illusory treatment goals. Imposing the idea of full "recovery," often equated with being "cured" (and not needing medications as a corollary) by patients and families, on partially refractory patients and families is cruel.

A less operationalized view sees recovery as a mind-set and process, not an end point. Recovery (or recovering) describes the process through which patients shed the patient label and develop identities (again) by which they are not defined by their illness or disability. Recovery means there is more to live for than visiting the doctor or the day program. In the broadest sense, recovery means being welcome in society and partaking of it (e.g., by voting), not being marginalized or hidden away. Even modest goals, such as reducing distress and reducing hospitalizations over the next 6 months, are valid steps in such recovery-oriented treatment.

 KEY POINT

One of the most grievous mistakes made in the care of patients with chronic illnesses, including schizophrenia, is to treat the chronic illness as if it were an acute illness. The goal for most acute illnesses is a *restitutio ad integrum*, a restoration to full health, a goal rarely achieved in schizophrenia. Patients (and their families) need to learn how to live with symptoms instead of waiting for the medicine to "kick in." A useful conception of recovery is having a meaningful and fulfilled life with, or even despite, an illness.

ADDITIONAL RESOURCES

Article

Carpenter Jr. WT. Evidence-based treatment for first-episode schizophrenia [editorial]? *Am J Psychiatry.* 2001;158: 1771–1773.—An important editorial highlighting the hard-to-ignore evidence base supporting antipsychotic maintenance treatment to reduce the otherwise almost inevitable relapse risk in schizophrenia.

Guidelines

So I do not appear biased, two treatment guidelines from different parts of the world:
American Psychiatric Association Practice Guidelines. Practice guideline for the treatment of patients with schizophrenia, 2nd ed. *Am J Psychiatry.* 2004;161(2 Suppl):1–56.

Royal Australian and New Zealand College of Psychiatrists Clinical Practice Guidelines Team for the Treatment of Schizophrenia and Related Disorders. Royal Australian and New Zealand College of Psychiatrists clinical practice guidelines for the treatment of schizophrenia and related disorders. *Aust N Z J Psychiatry.* 2005;39:1–30.

Antipsychotics— Overview

Essential Concepts

- All antipsychotics share varying degrees of dopamine-2 (D_2) blockade as the presumed main mechanism of action. Primary symptom targets of antipsychotics are positive symptoms (disorganization, delusions, and hallucinations) and agitation, with questionable efficacy for negative symptoms.
- Antipsychotics are grouped into first-generation antipsychotics—typical or conventional antipsychotics, which are all characterized by extrapyramidal symptom (EPS) liability—and second-generation antipsychotics (with reduced EPS risk, hence "atypical" antipsychotics). However, the second-generation antipsychotics (currently, aripiprazole, clozapine, olanzapine, paliperidone, quetiapine, risperidone, ziprasidone) should not be considered interchangeable, as patients might respond differently to each drug in this class.
- The main risks for first-generation antipsychotics are neurologic side effects (dystonias, akathisia, parkinsonism, and tardive dyskinesia); for most second-generation antipsychotics, metabolic problems (weight gain, dyslipidemia, and hyperglycemia) have emerged as major problems in management.
- First- and second-generation antipsychotics are about equally effective for nonrefractory patients with schizophrenia. For more refractory patients, olanzapine and, in particular, clozapine have shown the best efficacy.
- Clozapine has minimal to no EPS liability and is the most effective antipsychotic. However, its clinical use is limited to refractory patients because of serious side effects, including metabolic problems and agranulocytosis [which requires mandated white blood count (WBC) monitoring].

"The greater the ignorance, the greater the dogmatism."
—*Sir William Osler, Father of Modern Medicine, 1849-1919*

All currently marketed antipsychotics block D_2 receptors, albeit with different affinities. Side-effect differences can be predicted from the degree of D_2 is blockade (the more tightly bound to D_2 is the antipsychotic, the higher the risk for EPS) and the selectivity (histamine receptor binding is associated with sedation and weight gain, anticholinergic receptor binding with anticholinergic side effects, and adrenergic blockade with orthostatic hypotension). Clozapine and quetiapine are the antipsychotics with the least "tightness" of binding to D_2 (i.e., fastest dissociation from the receptor) and hence are the least likely to cause EPS, even at high doses (Kapur and Seeman, 2001). All antipsychotics are full D_2 antagonists with the exception of aripiprazole, which is a partial agonist at D_2.

One word on nomenclature: First-generation (or conventional) antipsychotics (FGAs) are old medications that were approved in the 1950s and 1960s. All are effective, and all cause EPS. FGAs are also referred to as "typical" antipsychotics to differentiate them from the "atypical" antipsychotic, clozapine, which was the first antipsychotic that did not cause EPS, hence "atypical." Its value was only recognized and proved in a seminal trial in 1988 when Kane showed superior efficacy in treatment-refractory patients over typical antipsychotics. Since then, other atypicals (or second-generation antipsychotics, SGAs) have been marketed, beginning with risperidone in 1994. Antipsychotic is the term preferred over neuroleptic.

◆ KEY POINT

A broad definition of "atypicality" denotes the absence of extrapyramidal side effects. More narrow definitions include the absence of hyperprolactinemia and broadened efficacy for negative symptoms. A neuroleptic is considered typical if it causes EPS at usual clinical doses (which is what you would expect from a "neuroleptic"—a "neuron-grabber").

For most antipsychotics, once-a-day dosing would be appropriate with regard to efficacy because the serum half-life of the antipsychotic does not reflect drug action on the brain. Ziprasidone is nevertheless usually administered twice daily (it is also the only antipsychotic that should be taken with food). Quetiapine, olanzapine, and clozapine are sometimes given more than once a day because of tolerability (or to take advantage of their sedating properties in acute settings), but nightly dosing works for most patients. The safe starting dose and the rapidity of titration depend on the clinical situation (e.g., age, gender, ethnicity, first-episode vs. multiepisode patient, acute vs. maintenance treatment phase). As a rule of thumb, start at the low end of the dose range for outpatients and increase the dose slowly. More aggressive dosing is possible in supervised inpatient settings.

FIRST-GENERATION ANTIPSYCHOTICS

The FGAs can be broadly classed into low-potency antipsychotics, medium-potency antipsychotics, and high-potency agents. The prototype of a low-potency FGA is chlorpromazine (brand name Thorazine), the first antipsychotic approved by the Food and Drug Administration (FDA) in 1954. Low-potency FGAs are not selective for the dopamine receptor; sedation, orthostatic hypotension, and anticholinergic side effects, as well as metabolic problems, are problematic. Haloperidol and fluphenazine are high-potency agents, which are highly selective for the D_2 receptor; predictably, side effects are largely restricted to the motor system. The medium-potency FGA, perphenazine, has a side-effect profile that falls in-between chlorpromazine and haloperidol with regard to EPS and sedation. Perphenazine has returned as an interesting antipsychotic choice after its good efficacy and tolerability were demonstrated in the Clinical Antipsychotic Trials of Intervention Effectiveness (CATIE; see Chapter 14 for more information on the seminal CATIE trial) in which it was chosen as the FGA comparator medication.

KEY POINT

For antipsychotic efficacy, about 65% of (striatal) D_2 receptors need to be blocked. Pushing the dose of tightly bound antipsychotics, such as all FGAs, beyond this point will not increase efficacy but will merely lead to EPS once a threshold of 80% occupancy is exceeded (Farde et al., 1988).

There is no advantage to switch between FGAs for better efficacy since they all share the same mechanism of D_2 blockade. The dosing of FGAs (Table 11.1; but not of SGAs) can be

TABLE 11.1. Dosing of Selected First-Generation Antipsychotics

	CPZ-Eq[a] (mg/day)	Typical Dose Range[b] (mg/day)
Low-potency		
Chlorpromazine	100	300–1000
Mid-potency		
Loxapine	10	30–100
Molindone	10	30–100
Perphenazine	10	16–64[c]
High-potency		
Trifluoperazine	5	15–50
Fluphenazine	2	5–20
Haloperidol	2	5–20

[a]CPZ-Eq, chlorpromazine dose equivalents.
[b]Dosing range is for chronic patients; first-episode patients require dosing at the lower end of the range.
[c]Clinical Antipsychotic Trials of Intervention Effectiveness (CATIE) dose range 8–32 mg/day; mean dose was 20 mg/day.
Adapted from Updated PORT Guideline (Lehman AF, Kreyenbuhl J, Buchanan RW, et al. The Schizophrenia Patient Outcomes Research Team (PORT): Updated treatment recommendations 2003. *Schizophr Bull.* 2004;30:193–217).

based on chlorpromazine equivalents (CPZ-Eq) as a guideline. Pushing the dose of FGAs reliably increases EPS but does not translate into further efficacy; it is not a good strategy to increase FGAs beyond recommended CPZ-Eq. Instead, use the "neuroleptic threshold," which is the point at which you just begin to see EPS (and which corresponds to 80% D_2 occupancy), to determine the optimal dose; exceeding the patient's neuroleptic threshold does not increase efficacy (McEvoy et al., 1991). The major long-term morbidity concern with FGAs is tardive dyskinesia. Haloperidol and fluphenazine have the advantage of being available as long-acting depot injections (the only other antipsychotic available as a long-acting injectable in the United States is risperidone); Table 11.2 presents dosing equivalencies.

TABLE 11.2. Dosing Equivalencies for Long-Acting Antipsychotics

Risperidone Consta 25 mg IM q2 weeks = 2 mg daily oral dose
Haloperidol decanoate 50 mg IM q4 weeks = 5 mg daily oral dose
Fluphenazine decanoate 6.25 mg IM q2 weeks = 5 mg daily oral dose

TIP

I suggest that you become familiar with at least one from each group of the FGAs. Be very familiar with the high-potency haloperidol because of its known efficacy and toxicities and availability for parenteral use (in the emergency department and the medical hospital). Medium-potency agents (e.g., perphenazine) have become an interesting treatment choice again. The occasional patient still takes chlorpromazine, and it can be a useful adjunctive option (also for second-line use in the emergency department). I do not prescribe pimozide, thioridazine, and mesoridazine because I think safer options are available (see Chapter 13).

SECOND-GENERATION ANTIPSYCHOTICS

Following clozapine as the prototype of an atypical antipsychotic, risperidone became the first in a series of antipsychotics with added serotonin 5-HT_2 antagonism after it was noted that this modification reduced neurologic side effects. All SGAs share this property and are thus 5-HT_2-D_2 antagonists. Risperidone is a first-line antipsychotic with known efficacy (at least comparable to FGAs) and known side effects (low EPS risk at typical doses below 6 mg/day but with clear EPS if you use higher doses). It has the advantage of being available as an injectable that can be given every 2 weeks. Compared to haloperidol, risperidone is more effective in preventing relapse in multiepisode patients (Csernansky et al., 2002). The active risperidone metabolite 9-hydroxyrisperidone was renamed paliperidone and is newly marketed in a formulation for once-daily use.

Olanzapine is sometimes effective when other antipsychotics are not, and olanzapine would be my first-line agent were it not for its higher liability for weight gain and diabetes. The CATIE results and other trials (Volavka et al., 2002) suggest that doses higher than the 20-mg FDA-approved dose (i.e., 30 mg or even 40 mg) have added efficacy compared to other antipsychotics except clozapine. I always suggest olanzapine to patients who had an insufficient response to other antipsychotics, before moving on to clozapine (see Chapter 25). Other than the well-recognized metabolic problems with olanzapine, sedation is a second factor that can prohibit the use of olanzapine if patients feel "drugged" all day.

Quetiapine and ziprasidone are effective antipsychotics, although doubt lingers about their efficacy in more refractory patients. For both drugs, dosing has not been worked out well, and doses higher than the FDA-approved doses (800 mg for quetiapine, and 160 mg for ziprasidone) are often given. However, the safety of these doses has not been studied. Ziprasidone is probably the safest antipsychotic regarding metabolic liability, and it causes sedation only rarely. Instead, activation and insomnia can occur, which may be treated with benzodiazepines. Quetiapine can be rather sedating and has anticholinergic like side effects (from its adrenergic properties).

Aripiprazole is an interesting antipsychotic in that it is the only partial dopamine agonist (with approximately 30% activity compared to dopamine) on the market in the United States. Partial agonists have the property of providing a ceiling of dopamine blockade; you cannot completely shut down dopamine transmission. This receptor-binding profile is probably responsible for fairly good tolerability—many of my patients prefer aripiprazole over other antipsychotics they have been on, as they do not seem to get the neuroleptic-induced dysphoria that characterizes excessive D_2 blockade. However, akathisia restlessness, activation, and insomnia can be problematic side effects, all of which are manageable with benzodiazepines. The efficacy question remains somewhat open, as aripiprazole was not included in CATIE. Note the very long half-life of 72 hours: Changes will become apparent 2 weeks after the dose increase; there is no need to "push the dose" during an acute admission. There is another reason that pushing the dose is probably unnecessary for many patients: 15 mg per day occupies almost all dopamine receptors (tightly); higher doses cannot change the intrinsic agonist/antagonist ratio for this partial agonist. The registration trials have found no added benefit from 20 or 30 mg doses. Table 11.3 details typical dosing ranges of SGAs, as well as those for refractory patients.

Clozapine

Clozapine is psychiatry's specialty drug, and it is our most effective, but also our most difficult to use, antipsychotic. Because it can cause agranulocytosis, a drug-based case registry is in place in the United States and many other countries, and patients have to submit to regular blood work. The agranulocytosis risk is but one potentially serious side effect, which leads many patients and psychiatrists to forgo a clozapine trial.

TABLE 11.3. Dosing of Second-Generation Antipsychotics

	Typical Dose Range (mg/day)		Refractory Patients[a] (mg/day)	
Aripiprazole	10–20		20–40	(30[b])
Clozapine[c]	200–300 ng/mL		>350 ng/mL	(900[b])
Olanzapine	7.5–30	(20[d])	30–40	(20[b])
Quetiapine	200–800	(543[d])	800–1200	(800[b])
Risperidone	2–8	(4[d])	8–12	(16[b])
Paliperidone[e]	3–9 (?)		9–15 (?)	(15[b])
Ziprasidone	80–160	(113[d])	160–320	(160[b])

[a]Only olanzapine has been shown to have advantages at higher doses. The safety of higher doses than FDA-approved doses has not been established.
[b]FDA-approved maximum daily dose.
[c]Dosing based on clozapine plasma levels (VanderZwaag et al., 1996). Maximum FDA approved daily oral dose is 900 mg, which can be insufficient to reach sufficient plasma levels.
[d]Average daily modal dose in CATIE.
[e]Newly released January 2007; starting dose 6 mg daily; effective doses 3–15 mg.

Clozapine is clearly indicated for patients who are treatment refractory (see Chapter 25). Other reasons you might want to use clozapine include sensitivity to motor side effects and tardive dyskinesia. Because clozapine can reduce suicidality and violence, you should also strongly consider it in those cases (Meltzer et al., 2003). "Softer" indications where clozapine might help are patients with comorbid substance use problems and those with psychogenic polydipsia.

To mitigate the risk from agranulocytosis, clozapine can only be dispensed if a patient is registered with a clozapine case registry and submits to regular blood draws. Before starting clozapine the WBC and absolute neutrophil count (ANC) need to be above an acceptable cutoff (WBC >3500/mm^3 and ANC >2000/mm^3). Should leukopenia/granulocytopenia develop during treatment, treatment either has to be monitored more frequently (for mild leukopenia/granulocytopenia), interrupted (for moderate leukopenia/granulocytopenia), or discontinued (for severe leukopenia/agranulocytosis) without the possibility of a rechallenge. Leukopenia occurs in 3% of cases. The risk for agranulocytosis is about 0.8% in the first year, highest during the first few months of treatment, but never returning to zero. Consistent with this nonlinear agranulocytosis risk the WBC and ANC are monitored weekly for 6 months, then every other week for 6 months, then every 4 weeks indefinitely as long as the patient continues on clozapine. With this blood-monitoring schedule, the risk of dying from agranulocytosis is low (obviously monitoring alone does not prevent bone marrow toxicity; it just detects it early enough so clozapine can be discontinued and patients can be monitored and treated). Some patients are not eligible for clozapine because of habitually low WBC counts, in which case you could add lithium to increase the WBC above the required threshold.

Seizures, syncope, and oversedation are the most pressing concerns when starting clozapine. A slow titration adjusted for tolerability is key. It is usually unnecessary to pretreat patients with an antiepileptic drug unless you think the patient has an increased seizure risk (e.g., organic brain injury). Benzodiazepines should be avoided with clozapine, particularly in this initial treatment phase because of the potential for severe interactions (resulting in death). Myocarditis is a problem that is not usually associated with antipsychotics but that is clearly described with clozapine. A high index of suspicion is necessary in patients who complain about fatigue, chest pain, or palpitations after starting clozapine.

The long-term management of clozapine is similar to other SGAs. However, weight gain and metabolic problems are often pronounced and must be taken into account when reviewing the risks and benefits of long-term clozapine treatment (Henderson et al., 2000).

ADDITIONAL RESOURCES

Book

Rosenbaum JF, Arana GW, Hyman SE, et al. *Handbook of psychiatric drug therapy.* 5th ed. Philadelphia: Lippincott Williams & Wilkins; 2005.—You need one book on psychopharmacology; I still use this one (Dr. Rosenbaum happens to be the chief of psychiatry of my department).

Article

Kontos N, Querques J, Freudenreich O. The problem of the psychopharmacologist. *Academic Psychiatry.* 2006;30: 218–226.— Mandatory reading if you consider yourself a "psychopharmacologist" after reading this chapter.

Antipsychotics—Motor Side Effects

Essential Concepts

- Motor side effects associated with antipsychotic treatment include acute extrapyramidal syndromes (acute dystonic reaction, akathisia, parkinsonism) and long-term complications [tardive dyskinesia (TD)].
- The *sine qua non* of akathisia is subjective restlessness with objective manifestations becoming apparent with increasing severity, possibly leading to bad outcomes (suicide attempts, nonadherence).
- Consider subtle forms of parkinsonism in blunted and slowed patients.
- TD can occur with all antipsychotics and treatment options are limited. The best option is to switch to an antipsychotic with less TD liability.
- Neuroleptic-induced dysphoria (NID) can lead to discontinuation of antipsychotic medication.
- Neuroleptic malignant syndrome (NMS) is a potentially fatal neurologic emergency characterized by a triad of fever, lead-pipe rigidity, and mental status changes.

> "Never mistake motion for action."
> —*Ernest Hemingway, Nobel Prize for literature 1954, 1899–1961*

Although neuroleptic-induced motor disorders are more common with first-generation antipsychotics (FGAs), they can occur with any antipsychotic. These iatrogenic motor disorders are considered extrapyramidal side effects (EPS) as they result from dopamine blockade in the posterior part of the basal ganglia (the motor loop). The distressing nature of EPS can lead patients to discontinue antipsychotic treatment, and permanent damage to the basal ganglia may occur, resulting in irreversible movements.

TIP

A motor examination can easily be done as part of any routine office visit. The key is to observe the patient sitting, talking, and walking. Look for evidence of tremor, bradykinesia, restlessness, or abnormal movements and specifically ask about inner sense of restlessness. To look for tremor, ask patients to hold out their hands, and examine for increased tone and cogwheeling at every visit. For simplicity, motor findings can be considered part of your mental status examination (MSE) and noted there.

ACUTE DYSTONIC REACTION

An acute dystonic reaction (ADR; involuntary, intermittent, sustained muscle contractions) is an early-onset EPS and can occur after a single dose of an antipsychotic. Half of cases occur within 2 days of starting treatment and almost all within 1 week. While an ADR is much more likely with high-potency FGAs, this side effect can occur with all antipsychotics, including clozapine.

KEY POINT

The acute onset of involuntary, sustained muscle contractions (dystonias) in the right setting (within a few days of starting an antipsychotic) should suggest an ADR.

Patients complain about "cramping," their "heads turning," problems with their eyes "rolling back," or a "thick" or protruding tongue. More dramatic manifestations, such as opisthotonus (body arching), torticollis, oculogyric crises (eyes rolling backward), or trismus (lockjaw), can occur. Patients can be distressed and overwhelmed with anxiety, but are not confused. Although distressing, dystonia is usually not dangerous except in cases of laryngeal–pharyngeal dystonia, which can result in respiratory compromise.

The clinical presentation of an ADR is usually acute and dramatic, and the diagnosis should not be difficult. Treatment with parenteral benztropine or diphenhydramine is highly effective.

TIP

If there is no response to treatment as usual, consider other etiologies. Phenylcyclohexylpiperidine (PCP) intoxication can cause dystonia and cocaine exacerbates drug-induced dystonias. Although rare, anticholinergics can be misused, and patients may fake an ADR to obtain them.

ADR is preventable by giving prophylactic anticholinergics to high-risk patients. Do not forget to discharge patients who had an acute dystonic reaction in the emergency department (ED) with a brief course of an anticholinergic. If no further antipsychotic treatment is planned, 2 or 3 days of benztropine (Cogentin) 1 or 2 mg bid or diphenhydramine (Benadryl) 25 to 50 qid is sufficient. I have seen patients return to the ED the next day with another episode of ADR because they did not receive prophylaxis.

AKATHISIA

Akathisia literally means "unable to sit still." It is an extremely unpleasant sense of inner restlessness with the desire to move about to relieve tension. As akathisia becomes more severe, you can observe the motor restlessness as patients may pace around, jiggle their feet, or be unable to sit and watch television for more than a few minutes at a time. It is one of the acute side effects, and I expect it to occur early in the course of treatment, sometimes after the first dose. Although FGAs, particularly high-potency antipsychotics like haloperidol or fluphenazine, can easily bring on akathisia, higher doses of second-generation antipsychotics can also cause it. The antipsychotics least likely to cause akathisia include quetiapine and clozapine.

The diagnosis of akathisia is usually straightforward. In the right clinical setting (i.e., after initiation of an antipsychotic), you should be alert for evidence of motor restlessness and always ask about an inner sense of restlessness. Some patients are objectively restless but deny the subjective component. In these circumstances I prefer to treat presumptively for akathisia. However, a diagnostic dilemma can occur when agitation in a very psychotic patient is either due to akathisia, requiring a reduction in antipsychotic treatment, or psychotic agitation, when increased treatment is needed.

Akathisia is not a side effect that patients should have to live with in the long run. If possible, lower the antipsychotic and hope the akathisia resolves. Otherwise, you might have to switch antipsychotics. Whatever you do, always treat akathisia symptomatically as well. Beta-blockers are considered the treatment of choice, and patients should be followed closely after initiation in case higher doses are required (start with propranolol 10 mg tid and titrate upward). Other effective medication classes include anticholinergics and benzodiazepines and, more recently, mirtazapine. In nonurgent cases I usually try to lower the antipsychotic dose while temporarily adding a benzodiazepine (e.g., clonazepam 1 mg bid).

 TIP

Akathisia can be very acute and severe. In a peracute case (which is an emergency), 10 mg diazepam brings instant relief. Even in less urgent cases, initiate treatment for akathisia and have the patient come for a follow-up in a few days to adjust the dose for efficacy.

PARKINSONISM

In its extreme form, parkinsonism is difficult to miss: Patients can be observed shuffling along the corridor, almost falling, without arm swing. During a visit to your office, they may sit with their mouth open, drool, have a coarse resting tremor, or need help getting out of the chair. Parkinsonism is usually symmetrical in the drug-induced form and is characterized by a triad of tremor, rigidity, and akinesia/bradykinesia. Subtle manifestations, however, are easy to overlook or misdiagnose, such as an apparent lack of facial expression being described as "blunted affect" and attributed to negative symptoms instead of the masked facies of parkinsonism. Signs and symptoms of parkinsonism usually appear within the first month of treatment and, as this side effect is often dose-related, reducing the dose of antipsychotic may solve the problem. If not, anticholinergic medications can be used, but attempts should be made to taper them after 3 months (see Chapter 27 for a more detailed discussion of why).

TARDIVE DYSKINESIA

The most feared, long-term (hence "tardive," which means late) consequence of treatment with dopamine-blocking agents is TD, a potentially irreversible movement disorder characterized by involuntary, choreiform movements. Less common, tardive akathisia or tardive dystonia are seen.

 KEY POINT

The risk for developing TD with FGAs is estimated to be 5% per year for the first few years of treatment in young adults. The risk is much higher for older patients (at least 25% per year). The risk for most second-generation antipsychotics is severalfold lower, albeit not zero (0.8% per year; Correll et al., 2004). Clozapine has the least TD liability.

Depending on the population, you can expect to find a TD prevalence of around 20%. This suggests two possibilities: (a) not all patients are at risk for TD (they are somehow protected biologically) and/or (b) TD can remit (which occurs in at least 5% of patients). One long-term study of 20 years found that most patients had TD at some point during the course of their illness and it remains of concern to all patients. It is also notable that abnormal movements were present in 10% of patients with schizophrenia who had never been exposed to antipsychotic medications (Gervin et al., 1998), suggesting that some cases of presumed drug-induced TD might be from the disease process itself. All these studies suggest that TD is a dynamic disorder, with the natural course interacting with antipsychotics in susceptible individuals. Risk factors for TD include age (older patients), female gender, and a history of early EPS.

Clinical Picture

Tardive movements from antipsychotics are typically choreiform (rapid and irregular), although athetoid (slow and writhing) or even dystonic movements (more sustained postures) are sometimes seen. Movements can be confined to the face (e.g., tongue protrusions, chewing movements, eye blinking, or "grimacing"), but other areas can also be affected.

Patients may seem to be moving their fingers as if playing the piano or truncal involvement can give patients the appearance of "dancing." Most cases of TD are mild with a waxing and waning course, and some (around 5%) even remit spontaneously despite ongoing treatment. Severely afflicted patients can be incapacitated by constant, severe movements that interfere with talking, eating, breathing (respiratory TD affecting the diaphragm), or walking.

Diagnosis

It requires much experience to correctly delineate the precise nature of the movements or recognize subtle TD (which can appear volitional—see epigraph to this chapter). TD is only one of many movement disorders to be considered (Table 12.1); get a neurologist to help sort it out. Note that antipsychotics can mask TD, which may become apparent only when reducing the dose. When antipsychotics are stopped, withdrawal dyskinesias can occur for several weeks, but they should eventually remit.

Once you have made the clinical diagnosis of TD, you can use the abnormal involuntary movement scale (AIMS) (see SCALE CARD AIMS in Appendix B) to record and follow the severity of the abnormal movements.

TABLE 12.1. Differential Diagnosis of Tardive Dyskinesia

Old age (edentulous patients; orobuccal dyskinesias of old age)
Meige syndrome
Blepharospasm
Stereotypies and dyskinesias of (never-treated) schizophrenia
Neurologic syndromes
    Choreas (e.g., Huntington's disease)
    Fahr's syndrome (idiopathic basal ganglia calcification)
    Wilson's disease
    Dystonias
    Tourette's syndrome or other tic disorders
    Restless leg syndrome
Toxins
Medications
Post anoxic or post encephalitis
Hypoparathyroidism
Systemic lupus erythematosus
Central nervous system neoplasm

Treatment

The best treatment is prevention: Use the lowest possible dose of any antipsychotic, but particularly an FGA and minimize lifetime exposure; or strongly consider a second-generation antipsychotic with lower TD risk. Periodically reassess the need for antipsychotics. If TD should develop, decide (again) if an antipsychotic is clearly needed, and discontinue the antipsychotic if possible. Consider a switch to clozapine, which has the least likelihood of causing TD (it might even treat it). In all cases I add vitamin E (1600 IU/day) as soon as I notice TD, as this might prevent further worsening of symptoms. In well-established cases of TD, vitamin E has no effect (Adler et al., 1999).

 TIP

For obvious medicolegal reasons, document specifically that the patient's informed consent included a discussion of TD when discussing the need and choice for *any* antipsychotic. Clearly document your baseline assessment of motor problems (which might be present), and monitor regularly. I check for EPS every patient visit and note "no abnormal movements" in the MSE, but also fill out an AIMS every 6 to 12 months.

NEUROLEPTIC-INDUCED DYSPHORIA

NID, a rather distressing, and frequently overlooked, subjective side effect, is thought to be a variant of EPS (Voruganti and Awad, 2004). Patients may describe a sense of listlessness and lack of motivation occurring after the first dose of an antipsychotic and lasting several weeks. NID is likely the result of dopamine blockade not in the nigrostriatal motor pathway but in the nucleus accumbens, a key structure in reward and motivation pathways. NID is related to the concept of "subjective well-being on neuroleptics" and a risk factor for treatment discontinuation.

NEUROLEPTIC MALIGNANT SYNDROME

NMS can be regarded as a severe form of EPS with systemic manifestations. NMS develops almost always (in 96% of patients in one study) within 30 days of starting an antipsychotic, although it can also rarely occur even years after initiating neuroleptics. The clinical picture develops rapidly (hours to days) and resolves (barring complications) within 30 days. NMS is characterized by a classic triad of fever (in all cases), lead-pipe muscular rigidity, and mental status changes. Vital signs are unstable, and patients are diaphoretic. Laboratory values show an increased creatine phosphokinase (CPK) from widespread myonecrosis and an increase in white blood cells. Rarely, atypical presentations without rigidity are possible with second-generation antipsychotics. Clozapine can also cause NMS!

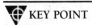 KEY POINT

NMS is a neurologic emergency. If you suspect NMS based on the classic triad of fever, lead-pipe rigidity, and mental status changes, hold all antipsychotics and refer the patient to the emergency room.

ADDITIONAL RESOURCES

Web Sites

http://www.nmsis.org—The NMS Information Service has many resources related to NMS, including a hotline for professionals.

http://www.mdvu.org—Contains much material about movement disorders, from Worldwide Education and Awareness for Movement Disorders (WE MOVE).

Antipsychotics—
Nonmotor Side Effects

Essential Concepts
- Nonmotor side effects of antipsychotics, such as sedation or weight gain, can reduce quality of life and lead to nonadherence.
- Metabolic side effects (i.e., diabetes mellitus and dyslipidemias) have become a major clinical concern and management issue, particularly for patients on second-generation antipsychotics.
- First-generation antipsychotics and risperidone reliably increase prolactin at usual doses, olanzapine at its higher dose range. Clozapine and quetiapine, ziprasidone, and aripiprazole are "prolactin-sparing."
- Assess side effects related to hyperprolactinemia clinically, as they are not associated with the degree of prolactin elevation. Typical side effects include erectile dysfunction and galactorrhea in males, and irregular or absent menses and galactorrhea in females.
- Antipsychotics can increase the risk for torsades de pointes if they prolong the QTc interval.
- Assess cardiac risk in all patients and monitor the electrocardiogram (ECG) in selected clinical situations (e.g., intravenous haloperidol use).
- Antipsychotics cause sexual side effects, and many patients are sexually active.

"Was mich nicht umbringt, macht mich härter."
("What does not kill me, makes me stronger.")
Friedrich Nietzsche, 1844–1900, Götzendämmerung

Nonmotor side effects are as important to patients as motor side effects and are probably in part responsible for nonadherence to second-generation antipsychotics—I think most patients would disagree with Nietzsche and not view side effects to antipsychotics as character building. Imagine you were asked to take a medicine long term that makes you feel sluggish for most of your waking hours. Knowing about and addressing these nonmotor side effects to increase "subjective well-being under neuroleptic treatment" are important to optimize adherence. Moreover, metabolic problems associated with antipsychotics (e.g., glucose intolerance or weight gain) are in part to blame for high rates of cardiovascular disease and premature mortality in patients with schizophrenia. In addition to this chapter, consult Chapter 21, which addresses weight gain and metabolic monitoring in more detail.

SEDATION

Sedation can be rather severe and lead to an inability to take the medication, as well as sleeping most of the day. For patients who have a problem with negative symptoms, this adds insult to injury. Clozapine, olanzapine, and quetiapine are clearly rather sedating for many patients, whereas aripiprazole and ziprasidone can lead to insomnia and are often poorly tolerated by chronic patients who have gotten used to the ataractic effects of their antipsychotic. Sedation depends on the degree to which histamine receptors are blocked by the antipsychotic.

With patients who have a "hangover" in the morning from a high nightly antipsychotic dose, you can try splitting up the dose or lowering the total daily dose. Short of changing the antipsychotic, coffee in the morning is sometimes sufficient (I think this is as effective as and safer than prescription stimulants or modafinil).

WEIGHT GAIN AND METABOLIC SIDE EFFECTS

Weight gain has always been a problem for patients taking psychotropics, but the second-generation antipsychotics have turned the spotlight even more on this issue. A very influential meta-analysis of weight gain propensity of antipsychotics has shown that not all antipsychotics are created equal when it comes to weight gain liability (Allison et al., 1999). Clozapine and olanzapine pose the biggest liability for weight gain, estimated to be more than 4 kg in 10 weeks of treatment, compared to 2 kg with risperidone. Ziprasidone was weight-neutral in this analysis, which did not include aripiprazole and quetiapine; molindone was associated with weight loss. In the Clinical Antipsychotic Trials of Intervention Effectiveness (CATIE), olanzapine led to a weight gain of 2 lb per month, risperidone and quetiapine had comparable weight gains of 0.5 lb per month, whereas patients assigned to ziprasidone or perphenazine lost weight.

As weight and body fat increases, insulin resistance increases, which can lead to a cluster of metabolic findings known as metabolic syndrome (syndrome X), that is, impaired glucose tolerance, hypertension, and dyslipidemia (see WELL CARD Metabolic Syndrome in Appendix C for more details). The relevance of the metabolic syndrome lies in its predictive value for cardiovascular disease and diabetes, making it all the more worrisome that 4 of 10 patients in CATIE had the metabolic syndrome (McEvoy et al., 2005). The typical patient develops diabetes as a late complication, in the setting of creeping but steady weight gain and increasing insulin resistance. Note, however, that in patients treated with second-generation antipsychotics, insulin resistance can develop in the absence of clinical obesity (Henderson et al., 2005), and patients can present with diabetic ketoacidosis as the first clinical sign of a metabolic problem. As a result, all second-generation antipsychotics carry a class warning about the possibility of diabetes and the need for clinical monitoring. Despite the class warning, the risk is not the same for all antipsychotics, and psychiatry's most effective antipsychotics, clozapine and olanzapine, carry the highest liability for the development of diabetes (American Diabetes Association, 2004). Clozapine and olanzapine also have the highest risk for increasing triglycerides (one of the parameters of the metabolic syndrome and a risk factor for pancreatitis if levels are very high). (See Chapter 21 for details on monitoring.)

HYPERPROLACTINEMIA AND SEXUAL SIDE EFFECTS

Recall from medical school that the prolactin inhibitory factor (PIF) turned out to be dopamine. Consequently, dopamine antagonists (i.e., antipsychotics) can increase prolactin. The first-generation antipsychotics risperidone and higher doses of olanzapine predictably lead to hyperprolactinemia; prolactin-sparing antipsychotics are clozapine, quetiapine, ziprasidone, and aripiprazole. Almost all patients treated with usual doses of risperidone will experience hyperprolactinemia (females relatively higher levels, but both sexes usually below 100 ng/mL). It is important to know that patients with increased prolactin levels do not automatically experience prolactin-related side effects; Table 13.1 presents a list of side

TABLE 13.1. Side Effects Related to Hyperprolactinemia

Decreased libido	In men: Erectile dysfunction
Anorgasmia	In women: Irregular menses or
Gynecomastia and	amenorrhea (with infertility)
galactorrhea	

effects. Although prolactin elevation is correlated with antipsychotic dose, clinical symptoms do not correlate with prolactin levels (Kleinberg et al., 1999).

For those patients who have symptoms attributable to hyperprolactinemia, I would first check the prolactin level and then consider switching to a prolactin-sparing antipsychotic. If the hyperprolactinemia is higher than you are comfortable with (e.g., above 200 ng/mL) or does not resolve after switching to a prolactin-sparing antipsychotic, further workup will be necessary to make sure your patient does not have a prolactinoma. The long-term effects of (asymptomatic) elevation of prolactin are unclear. However, prolactin-induced hypoestrogenemia can lead to osteoporosis, and I would monitor bone density in premenopausal women with antipsychotic-induced amenorrhea (Naidoo et al., 2003). For some women, hormone replacement therapy should be considered.

 TIP

Warn female patients with amenorrhea from antipsychotics that their menses (and fertility!) might return when they are switched to prolactin-sparing antipsychotics. Discuss contraception with your female patients of childbearing age.

CLINICAL VIGNETTE

I had known a female patient with schizophrenia and alcoholism for many years. A severe alcoholic, her adherence to antipsychotics was marginal at best, and she went in and out of detoxification units, homeless shelters, and psychiatric hospitals until long-acting risperidone led to a period of psychiatric stability followed by cessation of drinking. The patient did not have any clinical signs of hyperprolactinemia other than amenorrhea, which did not bother her. Because she was clinically stable, we decided together to continue risperidone. Her initial prolactin level (while on risperidone) was 147 ng/mL, which has remained stable for the past 2 years. Serial prolactin levels are useful to exclude a prolactinoma (where levels would rise).

Many patients struggle with loss of libido as a function of dopamine blockade and hyperprolactinemia. Sexual side effects of antipsychotics are usually missed, as nobody seems to ask but everybody assumes patients to be "asexual." This is untrue: Patients with schizophrenia are sexually active, and this means that female patients can get pregnant and that all patients are at risk for sexually transmitted diseases, including human immunodeficiency virus (HIV). It is worthwhile not to assume anything, so you should have a discussion about sexual topics with your patients. Simply ask: "Are you sexually active?" and take it from there.

Priapism is a potentially serious adverse reaction to antipsychotics with prominent α-1 blockade: risperidone, olanzapine, and clozapine. Warning signs are prolonged erections. Erectile dysfunction from antipsychotics might respond to a trial of sildenafil.

CARDIAC TOXICITY

Although rare, antipsychotics, particularly thioridazine, have been implicated in sudden death in several epidemiologic studies. Pimozide, although sometimes touted as the best treatment for delusional disorder, has calcium channel–blocking properties and should only be used if you monitor the ECG. Personally, I do not use thioridazine (or its metabolite mesoridazine) or pimozide because safer options that are as effective are available. Many emergency departments avoid droperidol because of (an admittedly controversial) black-box warning about QTc prolongation.

Antipsychotics cause arrhythmias via prolongation of the action-potential phase of the cardiac cycle, by delaying ventricular repolarization and thereby increasing the risk for torsades de pointes (a potentially deadly ventricular arrhythmia) (Glassman and Bigger, 2001). This effect on repolarization is reflected in a prolonged QTc interval on the ECG. The propensity to prolong the QTc interval is different for different antipsychotics, with thioridazine the clear winner (or loser, if you will). Ziprasidone can demonstrably increase QTc (by about 16 ms on average), but it is reassuring that

QTc prolongation greater than 500 ms is very rare and that there is no dose-related QTc prolongation. The latter is important because it suggests that overdoses or blocking the metabolism of ziprasidone should not increase cardiac risk beyond the small, expected QTc prolongation. Although the most conservative approach is to check and follow ziprasidone patients with an ECG, this is probably of little clinical benefit in healthy patients and, as far as I can tell, not routinely done. For outpatients, it makes sense to check an ECG in patients who are older or in those with cardiac risk factors (which your assessment should include, along with whether they take any other QTc-prolonging medications). Follow the ECG if you use intravenous haloperidol.

Medications with α-blocking properties (i.e., low-potency antipsychotics and clozapine) can cause orthostatic hypotension and need to be titrated at the beginning of treatment. Consider orthostasis if your patient complains about dizziness or even falls at home. Clozapine once again stands out with a particularly dangerous cardiac side effect, myocarditis, which can develop early in the course of treatment.

ANTICHOLINERGIC SIDE EFFECTS

Antipsychotics that are anticholinergic can be expected to cause a dry mouth, blurry vision, and constipation, but more serious side effects are possible (e.g., toxic megacolon). The low-potency first-generation antipsychotic chlorpromazine is strongly anticholinergic, as is clozapine. Paradoxically, clozapine can cause sialorrhea. Quetiapine can cause anticholinergic like side effects via adrenergic mechanisms, including constipation and dry mouth.

OTHER SIDE EFFECTS

With some older medications, eye problems can develop. Chlorpromazine can cause pigment changes affecting the retina (it also causes general pigmentation of the skin and photosensitivity), and thioridazine causes a pigmentary retinopathy at doses greater than 800 mg per day. The most relevant eye concern in our patient population is cataracts. Patients with schizophrenia have many risk factors for cataracts (e.g., smoking and diabetes), so it is not clear if medications are additional risk factors. The concern that quetiapine causes cataracts (which lead to mentioning the need for serial slit-lamp examinations in the package insert) is based on animal studies and has not been confirmed in humans; see Fraunfelder (2004) for a comment.

 TIP

Given the lack of eye care in general, it might not be a bad idea to refer your patients for a basic eye examination, as part of caring for them medically. To kill two birds with one stone (reduce your medicolegal liability and provide preventive eye care), I would encourage any patient who is going to take quetiapine *long term* to see an ophthalmologist.

Antipsychotics can increase the risk of seizures, with clozapine having the highest risk, followed by chlorpromazine. The risk increases with dose (or, rather, blood level), rapidity of dose escalation, and susceptibility of the brain (e.g., organic brain disease).

Antipsychotics are not nephrotoxic, and not usually hematotoxic or hepatotoxic. What this means is that routine blood work to check for renal function, blood cells, and liver function is usually neither necessary nor done. There are exceptions: Clozapine can lead to agranulocytosis, and many antipsychotics can lead to usually mild liver function test abnormalities at the start of treatment; chlorpromazine can be hepatotoxic, with cholestasis the typical finding.

ADDITIONAL RESOURCES

Article

Naber D, Karow A, Lambert M. Subjective well-being under the neuroleptic treatment and its relevance for compliance. *Acta Psychiatr Scand Suppl.* 2005;427:29–34.—An article that introduces the idea of "subjective well-being under neuroleptic treatment," a construct that brings back the importance of a patient's experience with the medication (including side effects).

Antipsychotics—Clinical Effectiveness

Essential Concepts

- A large clinical trial, Clinical Antipsychotic Trials of Intervention Effectiveness (CATIE), compared risperidone, olanzapine, quetiapine, and ziprasidone with perphenazine. Only 26% of subjects who entered this 18-month trial completed their assigned treatment, suggesting less-than-optimal effectiveness (efficacy and tolerability) of currently available antipsychotics.

- Antipsychotics are selected based on individualized risk–benefit assessments (balancing psychiatric stability with day-to-day tolerability and long-term medical morbidity, particularly cardiovascular risk). To find the best medication for a patient usually requires sequential trials in a collaborative manner.

- Include long-acting antipsychotics in the list of choices to routinely offer your patients, not only to those who refuse medications.

- Switching antipsychotics to reduce long-term cardiovascular risk can be an appropriate clinical decision, albeit at the risk of psychiatric instability.

"Plus ça change, plus c'est la même chose."
("The more things change,
the more they stay the same.")
—*Alphonse Karr, French critic, journalist, writer, editor of Les Guêpes where the epigram was published in 1849*

The arrival of second-generation antipsychotics (SGAs) in the 1990s led to great excitement among both patients and psychiatrists. Although this optimism might seem naïve and unbridled today, it is important to remember that psychiatric drug development had made little (some would say no) progress beyond chlorpromazine, even though the limits of dopamine antagonists, both in terms of efficacy and side effects (i.e., tardive dyskinesia), had become painfully clear. This changed with the publication of one of the truly seminal trials in psychiatry, the Kane trial (Kane et al., 1988), which showed that clozapine can be effective in patients who are refractory to first-generation antipsychotics (FGAs). In the following decade, SGAs other than clozapine became available for clinical use and became the treatment of choice for many patients in the United States.

However, almost all data supporting the superiority of SGAs had came from industry-sponsored drug trials, and some became convinced that the claims of superiority of SGAs were the result of comparing SGAs to what are today considered excessive haloperidol doses (Geddes et al., 2000). Others found somewhat better efficacy for some (clozapine, olanzapine, and risperidone), but not all, compared to FGAs, consistent with the heterogeneity of SGAs (Davis et al., 2003). Clinicians also started to notice that SGAs (while having a lower risk for tardive dyskinesia) had shifted the side-effect burden to metabolic problems.

CLINICAL ANTIPSYCHOTIC TRIALS OF INTERVENTION EFFECTIVENESS

To remedy this lack of independent and generalizable data, the National Institute of Mental Health (NIMH) decided to sponsor a large, randomized trial, CATIE, comparing the SGAs available at the time (olanzapine, quetiapine, risperidone; ziprasidone was added after the trial was at about the midway point; aripiprazole was not available) with each other and with a fairly low dose of the midpotency antipsychotic perphenazine (Phase I). In all, 1,493 patients were recruited from more than 50 representative sites in the United States and followed, double blind after randomization, for 18 months. The main outcome variable was all-cause discontinuation, a summary measure combining efficacy and tolerability. The focus of CATIE on effectiveness (to understand how a drug performs in real-world settings) is rather different than the typical pharmacologic efficacy trial (in which drug effects are studied under ideal conditions in homogeneous populations). CATIE patients who failed their initially assigned treatment because of lack of efficacy could go on to a second phase that included treatment with clozapine. The main results of Phase I were disappointing: Only 26% of subjects completed the trial on their initially assigned antipsychotic, pointing

TABLE 14.1. Lessons from Clinical Antipsychotic Trials of Intervention Effectiveness

---

- All antipsychotics have limitations in the real world with regard to efficacy, tolerability, or both; this leaves many patients unwilling to take them in the long run.
- Type and severity of side effects differ between SGAs; they should not be regarded as one class, and patients should have access to all of them to individualize their treatment since no single antipsychotic is optimal for all, or even most, patients.
- Olanzapine and clozapine are most effective, albeit at a high side-effect burden.
- Ziprasidone has the least weight and metabolic side-effect burden.
- Perphenazine's effectiveness and tolerability were comparable to SGAs and it deserves to be given a second look; however, the comparative tardive dyskinesia risk with perphenazine compared to SGAs was not addressed in CATIE.
- SGAs might be most useful for more symptomatic or refractory patients.

---

toward major problems with available antipsychotics (Lieberman et al., 2005). Phase II confirmed the superiority of clozapine over available SGAs (McEvoy et al., 2006). Some clinical lessons from CATIE are summarized in Table 14.1. Another randomized trial conducted in Europe, CUtLASS 1 (Cost Utility of the Latest Antipsychotic Drugs in Schizophrenia Study) similarly found older FGAs (in particular, one not available in the United States, sulpiride) as effective and as well tolerated as SGAs (Jones et al., 2006). In the end, the SGAs might not have been the major advance for all patients they were once hoped to be, and I think we will revisit the use of FGAs, particularly some midpotency FGAs.

CHOOSING ANTIPSYCHOTICS

Individual patients show marked differences in their clinical response and tolerability to any given antipsychotic. Because you cannot predict which medication is going to show the best benefit–risk ratio for individual patients, you will usually have to do sequential trials to empirically figure this out in collaboration with your patients. The side-effect profile can help narrow your initial choices; for example, for a patient who sleeps poorly, you might consider a more sedating antipsychotic first. For some patients, you can to take into account personal or family medical history; for example, for an overweight patient with a strong family history of diabetes, ziprasidone would be a logical first choice. For others, the preference of avoiding a particular side effect (e.g., any degree of possible weight gain) weighs heavily for or against a particular drug.

KEY POINT

For many patients, the best (i.e., most effective) long-term antipsychotic will represent a compromise between efficacy and tolerability. The only way of tailoring your antipsychotic treatment to your patient is by trial and error in the form of sequential trials.

Other, important variables that will influence your choice of medication and dose are the following:

- Age—Children and elderly patients require different antipsychotic doses. Children require relatively higher oral doses because of increased liver metabolism; and frail, geriatric patients at times very low doses.
- Gender—Female patients pose additional problems with family planning and side effects related to the reproductive system. The required antipsychotic dose is generally lower (Seeman, 2004).
- Ethnicity—Optimal antipsychotic doses might vary with ethnicity, in part from genetically determined differences in metabolism.

In patients who sabotage their own treatment and rehabilitation with frequent relapses due to nonadherence to antipsychotics, the mode of administration becomes as important as other considerations. I always include a long-acting antipsychotic as an excellent choice for all patients, given the chronic nature of the disease and the need for ongoing antipsychotics. If presented as one of the choices at the beginning of treatment, it becomes an easier sell when you become concerned about partial adherence.

 TIP

I offer a time-limited trial of a long-acting antipsychotic to all patients, including first-episode patients. This is not only an excellent clinical option but avoids the idea of getting punished with "a shot" if the patient "fails" oral medications.

SWITCHING ANTIPSYCHOTICS

Switching antipsychotics comes up regularly in the outpatient setting, as the typical patient is burdened with side effects from only partially effective medications. Many questions about switching are judgment calls with no obviously right or wrong answer: What symptom level should trigger a switch? Should you switch for nonpsychotic symptoms (negative or cognitive symptoms)? Should you switch elderly patients who have missed the atypical revolution because of the possibility of tardive dyskinesia as the brain ages? Should you switch because of increased cholesterol? The decision is difficult, and risk–benefit discussions should involve all parties affected by the switch, which is often not just the patient but also family members or care providers as well. Whenever possible, optimize the current antipsychotic first (e.g., assure maximal compliance and optimal dosage) before switching. In the CATIE sample (of treatment-experienced, chronic patients), those who did not switch (i.e., they were randomly assigned to the same antipsychotic they had entered the trial on) fared somewhat better than those who were assigned to switch (Essock et al., 2006).

These are common outpatient reasons for switching antipsychotics:

- Switching for ongoing, residual positive symptoms, particularly if they interfere with day-to-day functioning
- Switching for secondary negative symptoms (including sedation)
- Switching for distressing side effects that decrease quality of life (e.g., akathisia)
- Switching because of concerns about long-term medical morbidity (i.e., weight gain, diabetes, dyslipidemia) (see Chapter 21)
- Switching because of nonadherence (e.g., to a long-acting antipsychotic)

The question of switching to "the new medication" comes up invariably when a new antipsychotic enters the market. Help patients understand that medications (or medication switches) are at best part of the solution. In some patients you encounter the opposite problem. Even though you think a switch makes sense because of lack of efficacy, the family or group home does not want to rock the boat, according to the myth that "things could be worse."

TIP

The question to ask about the new drug is not how it is better, but rather how it is different. Do not promise a cure, but suggest that improvement in overall well-being without freedom from symptoms is probably a more realistic goal. In many patients, switching to reduce cardiovascular risk factors (as opposed to psychiatric efficacy) has become an important risk–benefit consideration.

The mechanics of switching are uncomplicated (and are often made more complicated than necessary), with the most conservative approach being never to leave patients uncovered (i.e., not dopamine-2 blocked) during a cross-titration to avoid acute withdrawal phenomena, including a withdrawal psychosis. As a general approach, I leave the old antipsychotic aboard at full dose, initiate the new antipsychotic and titrate it to its full therapeutic target dose quickly, overlap for 2 weeks, and only then start tapering the old antipsychotic. Modify this schema based on individual tolerability, but try to get the crossover done in 1 month to minimize environmental interference that could lead to clinical instability. Also, keep it simple to minimize room for medication error, and persist in switching over even if there is apparent improvement halfway through (to avoid the stalled-taper phenomenon).

CLINICAL VIGNETTE

A patient whom I "inherited" had been clinically stable on olanzapine for many years, without psychosis and had not required hospitalizations. Because he had developed the metabolic syndrome, the patient and his family, at the urging of the primary care physician, wanted his olanzapine switched to ziprasidone; a reasonable clinical decision, particularly because behavioral measures were unsuccessful in improving his health. Unfortunately, he became psychotic 1 month after the switch and required several hospitalizations over the course of 6 months, eventually stabilizing on olanzapine again.

Since relapse is a real risk even in patients who have been asymptomatic for many years, always discuss the risks, benefits, and alternatives (including no change) of any switch. A switch is rarely an emergency; you have time to get everybody aboard before the switch (unless you want to get the blame for a failed switch: "You never told us he could end up in the hospital again"). Recall that the psychotic relapse risk remains constant and does not decrease with time: Even a decade of stability does not ensure a relapse-free switch.

ADDITIONAL RESOURCES

Web Site

http://www.catie.unc.edu/schizophrenia/—This is the official CATIE Web site, which explains this complex study in more detail. A useful feature is a publication list.

Articles

Lieberman JA, Stroup TS, McEvoy JP, et al. Effectiveness of antipsychotic drugs in patients with chronic schizophrenia. *N Engl J Med.* 2005;353:1209–1223.—The landmark CATIE trial.

Lieberman JA. Comparative effectiveness of antipsychotic drugs. A commentary on: Cost Utility of the Latest Antipsychotic Drugs in Schizophrenia Study (CUtLASS 1) and Clinical Antipsychotic Trials of Intervention Effectiveness (CATIE) [editorial]. *Arch Gen Psychiatry.* 2006;63: 1069–1072.—Principal investigator of CATIE, Dr. Jeffrey Lieberman, summarizes in this editorial his current thinking about SGAs versus FGAs in the post-CATIE, post-CUtLASS 1 era.

15 ▼ Ancillary Medications

Essential Concepts

- Avoid antidepressants during acute episodes of psychosis, but consider antidepressants in patients with remitted schizophrenia who develop full, syndromal depression.
- Valproate is useful adjunctively in acute psychosis to decrease agitation. Its value in the long-term management of schizophrenia is less clear, except possibly in cases with chronic irritability or excitability.
- Lithium is not useful for psychosis per se, and it carries the risk of neurotoxicity when combined with antipsychotics.
- Carbamazepine is probably most useful (if at all) for patients with schizophrenia and neurologic problems.
- Benzodiazepines are useful for ancillary problems such as insomnia and anxiety disorders. They can be used to stave off relapse, instead of increasing antipsychotics.
- Anticholinergics should only be used short term because of impairment of memory.

> "At some point, you have to get off the sandbar and suggest some type of treatment to help those in distress."
> —*George B. Murray, MD, Massachusetts General Hospital*

As I have stated throughout the book, antipsychotics are not antischizophrenic medications; their main usefulness lies in reducing positive symptoms acutely and preventing psychotic relapse in the long run. Psychiatrists use medications from many other drug classes adjunctively to target side effects and nonpsychotic symptoms, admittedly often with limited evidence. After reading this chapter, read Chapter 17 to guard against prescribing too much, but be willing to try new treatments to help your patient, as Dr. Murray's dictum suggests.

ANTIDEPRESSANTS

Antidepressants are widely used in schizophrenia because dysphoria and depressive symptoms are common problems for patients. Although antidepressants seem like a good idea in this clinical scenario, their usefulness has never been clearly established. Much of the literature on antidepressants for schizophrenia stems from the era of first-generation antipsychotics and tricyclic antidepressants. The older literature suggests that tricyclic antidepressants added during an acute psychotic symptom exacerbation will in fact impede resolution of psychosis, whereas postpsychotic depressive episodes are helped with antidepressants, and some patients will relapse if antidepressants are discontinued. This field of inquiry is hampered by a high placebo-response rate to antidepressants, 50% in one study that compared sertraline with placebo in patients with remitted schizophrenia who had a depressive episode (Addington et al., 2002).

 TIP

Avoid antidepressants in acutely psychotic patients with schizophrenia; an antipsychotic alone will usually lead to resolution of depressive symptoms. Consider adding an antidepressant in the postpsychotic or stable period if a full depressive syndrome develops in otherwise remitted patients. Make sure you measure the severity of depression with a rating scale. (The specific Calgary Depression Scale for Schizophrenia, or CDSS, works satisfactorily, but I have found the patient-rated Beck Depression Inventory easy to use serially).

There is a small literature that selective serotonin reuptake inhibitors (SSRIs) can be a useful adjunct to treat negative symptoms (Rummel et al., 2005). The effect size is small, and I am unsure if you can truly see a clinical difference in most patients. Nevertheless, given the lack of good treatment options, a time-limited trial can be justified.

Recently, mirtazapine has been shown in a controlled trial to be rather effective for akathisia. Remember to follow a patient's weight if you prescribe mirtazapine for long-term use.

ANXIOLYTICS

Most psychiatrists who treat many patients with schizophrenia will agree with me that benzodiazepines are a very useful medication class for adjunctive use in patients with schizophrenia, both during the acute treatment phase and the chronic phase, even though very few pharmacology trials have been conducted. Table 15.1 gives indications for which a benzodiazepine could be considered. Note that benzodiazepines are a first-line treatment for catatonia. When you use benzodiazepines, keep in mind the possibility of impairing cognition (but also the deleterious effects of untreated anxiety on performance).

One of the few controlled trials of benzodiazepines for the treatment of schizophrenia found adding the benzodiazepine diazepam as effective as increasing the antipsychotic fluphenazine, in the case of the study, to stave off a psychotic relapse (Carpenter et al., 1999).

 TIP

If your patient experiences some stress and you are worried about a psychotic relapse, add diazepam (Valium), 10 mg up to three times per day, instead of increasing the antipsychotic (to avoid side effects related to higher antipsychotic doses).

Insomnia

Sleep problems are very common in schizophrenia. I think benzodiazepines are underused for insomnia, often at the expense of more risky approaches (e.g., the atypical antipsychotic

TABLE 15.1. Indications for Benzodiazepines in Schizophrenia

Acute agitation
Unspecific anxiety and specific anxiety syndromes
Early signs of psychotic relapse
Akathisia
Hostility and aggression
Insomnia
Catatonic symptoms

quetiapine). Benzodiazepines are one of the safest medications we have in our armamentarium. Although there is always the possibility of misuse with benzodiazepines, you figure out quickly whom to prescribe benzodiazepines to and whom not to. Of course, make sure that no specific sleep disorder is present. Common disorders are obstructive sleep apnea or simply poor sleep hygiene and sleep–wake cycle disturbances for which benzodiazepines are of little to no use. Some more-activating antipsychotics (e.g., ziprasidone) can cause insomnia, and adding a benzodiazepine at night remedies the problem. Insomnia can be a problem for patients who are used to sedating antipsychotics when they are switched to less-sedating antipsychotics.

CLINICAL VIGNETTE

Matthias suffers from schizophrenia with well-controlled positive symptoms but has difficulties getting around in the city because he avoids the subway ("people make me nervous"). Initially attributed to subtle paranoia and social uneasiness commonly seen in schizophrenia, you learn he also avoids escalators and bridges. On further questioning, he endorses clear and frequent panic attacks and avoidance of situations he fears could induce a panic attack. The addition of a benzodiazepine completely stops the panic attacks, and he is venturing out more easily in the city. Comorbid, syndromal anxiety disorders, in particular panic disorder, are not uncommon in schizophrenia and can be easily missed, yet are very treatable. Consider treating panic attacks even if they occur in response to paranoia.

MOOD STABILIZERS

Lamotrigine

Lamotrigine is one of the few medications that have shown some promise in controlled clinical trials as an add-on medication for patients with schizophrenia. I try it in patients with persistent psychosis, particularly if they have chronic dysphoria or dysthymia as well (remember, it is approved for bipolar depression, for which it has been shown to work). Clinical trials have used total daily doses of 200 to 400 mg. I have found lamotrigine to be one of the better-tolerated antiepileptic drugs used in psychiatry, with little sedation or weight gain. However, you must strictly follow titration guidelines to minimize the risk for Stevens–Johnson syndrome.

Lithium

Lithium alone is ineffective for the core symptoms of schizophrenia (Leucht et al., 2004). A trial of lithium is nevertheless reasonable in refractory cases with periodicity in the presentation or significant admixture of mood symptoms such as irritability with aggression. The risks from lithium use must be taken into consideration, particularly the higher side-effect burden and the risk of neuroleptic malignant syndrome (NMS) and other neurotoxic effects (e.g., delirium, increased extrapyramidal symptoms, or EPS) from combining lithium with antipsychotics. The lifetime risk for serious lithium toxicity is not negligible in complex patients, and the psychosocial situation has to be taken into account if one plans to use lithium for maintenance treatment of schizophrenia.

Valproate

Valproate is somewhat useful for the acute management of psychosis, although its role in the long-term management of schizophrenia is questionable. When valproate is combined with an antipsychotic, acutely psychotic patients become calmer more quickly than with the antipsychotic alone; however, both approaches lead to the same degree of improvement after several weeks of treatment. I think it is a common mistake to simply continue valproate with an outpatient if it was added in the hospital for faster behavioral control. For refractory and chronic irritability, valproate is commonly used (including by me), although I admit that the benefit of this approach is not well documented.

In my experience, valproate is not as well tolerated as many seem to think; sedation, worsened EPS, and weight gain are expectable problems (in addition to a host of potentially more severe problems such as pancreatitis). In women, take into account that valproate is associated with polycystic ovary syndrome (PCOS).

Carbamazepine and Oxcarbazepine

Apart from unclear efficacy for schizophrenia, the clinical use of carbamazepine and oxcarbazepine is limited by enzyme induction, more so for carbamazepine than with oxcarbazepine, leading to problems achieving sufficient antipsychotic drug levels. I consider them third-line add-on treatments unless there are electroencephalogram (EEG) abnormalities. Note bone marrow toxicity with carbamazepine (do not combine with clozapine) and hyponatremia with oxcarbazepine (particularly in elderly patients).

ANTICHOLINERGICS

Chronic use of anticholinergics is very problematic: They impair memory and complex attention, both of which are impaired in schizophrenia to begin with (see Chapter 27). Other concerns include worsening tardive dyskinesia and increasing the peripheral side-effect burden in the form of constipation or blurred vision. Some patients might misuse anticholinergics. The acute use of anticholinergic medications for a week or so (e.g., to prevent an adverse drug reaction, or ADR, in high-risk cases of young patients who receive first-generation antipsychotics) can be a reasonable clinical decision. In selected cases, a trial to eliminate the possibility of secondary negative symptoms from subtle EPS can be considered. However, the World Health Organization (WHO) in

TABLE 15.2. Dosing Guidelines for Anticholinergics, Diphenhydramine, and Amantadine

Agent	Benztropine Equivalents	Typical Dose Range	Max Dose/day
Benztropine (Cogentin)[a]	1 mg	0.5–2 bid	6 mg
Biperiden (Akineton)[a]	2 mg	1–2 bid/tid	16 mg
Trihexyphenidyl (Artane)	3.5 mg	2–5 bid/tid	15 mg
Procyclidine (Kemadrin)	?	2.5–5 tid	30 mg
Diphenhydramine (Benadryl)[a]	30 mg	25–50 tid/qid	400 mg
Amantadine (Symmetrel)	N/A	100 bid/tid	300 mg
For comparison:			
Chlorpromazine	300 mg		
Clozapine	50–100 mg		

[a]Available for intramuscular use in the United States.

a consensus statement strongly recommends against the routine, prophylactic use of anticholinergics. Instead, anticholinergics should only be used in cases in which parkinsonism actually develops and other measures prove ineffective (World Health Organization Heads of Centres Collaborating in WHO Co-ordinated Studies on Biological Aspects of Mental Illness, 1990). Even in those cases, attempts to discontinue the anticholinergic after 3 months are recommended. If EPS develop with an antipsychotic, try to switch to an antipsychotic that does not require the chronic use of anticholinergics. Alternatively, you could try adding amantadine instead (which might even have a positive effect on weight); Table 15.2 presents dosing guidelines.

ADDITIONAL RESOURCES

Article

Goff DC, Freudenreich O, Evins AE. Augmentation strategies in the treatment of schizophrenia. *CNS Spectr.* 2001;6: 904–911.—A review of augmentation strategies by the Massachusetts General Hospital Schizophrenia Program.

Drug Interactions

Essential Concepts
- All antipsychotics are metabolized to varying degrees by the hepatic cytochrome P450 (CYP450) isoenzymes 3A4, 2D6, and 1A2. Some have additional non-P450 metabolism, which lowers the risk for drug interactions by providing alternative pathways if major pathways are inhibited.
- Because 3A4 metabolizes the bulk of antipsychotics, inducers and inhibitors of 3A4 are important clinically.
- Smoking increases the metabolism of 1A2-dependent antipsychotics, requiring dose adjustment for olanzapine and clozapine.
- Although antipsychotics are generally safe even with excessive drug serum levels, pimozide, mesoridazine/thioridazine (cardiac toxicity), and clozapine (seizures and hypotension) are exceptions.
- Some drug interactions problems are "hidden" in that they merely increase the statistical risk factors for later morbidity (e.g., for tardive dyskinesia or diabetes).
- Antipsychotic serum drug levels are not useful routinely, but rather in clinical situations in which you want to confirm that a patient is at the extremes of drug levels.

> "I beseech you, in the bowels of Christ, think
> it possible you may be mistaken."
> —Oliver Cromwell, Lord protector of England, 1599-1658

"I don't think this is related to my medicine," you hear yourself telling your patient. Never dismiss a patient's complaint about a side effect, but consider the possibility that you are wrong and the patient is right, possibly because of a hitherto unrecognized drug interaction (Cromwell puts the patient's complaint in more dramatic language).

In this chapter, I focus mostly on drug metabolism, particularly the all-important CYP450 enzyme system that does the bulk of metabolism for psychotropics, including antipsychotics, and how it relates to serum drug levels. Renal excretion and plasma binding are generally not a clinical issue with antipsychotics.

ANTIPSYCHOTIC DRUG METABOLISM

Antipsychotics are mainly metabolized by the hepatic CYP450 enzyme system, but other systems, like the phase II glucuronidation enzyme system (uridine glucuronosyl transferase, or UGT), contribute to the deactivation of antipsychotics. For antipsychotic metabolism, the most important cytochrome isoenzymes are 3A4, 2D6, and 1A2. Consult Table 16.1 for the main metabolic pathways for commonly used antipsychotics.

TABLE 16.1. Antipsychotic Metabolic Pathways

Relevant Metabolite	CYP450 Metabolism	Alternative Metabolism
First-generation antipsychotics		
Haloperidol	HP^{+a}	**3A4, 2D6** Glucuronidation
Fluphenazine	7-OH-FLU^b	**2D6**
Perphenazine	None known	**2D6**
Second-generation antipsychotics		
Aripiprazole	None active	**3A4, 2D6**
Clozapine	nor-CLZ^c	**1A2, 3A4,** 2C19, (2D6)
Olanzapine	None active	**1A2,** (2D6, 2C19?) **Glucuronidation**
Quetiapine	None relevant	**3A4,** (2D6)
Risperidone	9-OH-RSP^d	**2D6,** 3A4
Ziprasidone	None relevant	**3A4** (33%) **Aldehyde oxidase** (66%)

Main metabolizing enzymes in **bold**.
^{a}HP+ is likely a neurotoxic metabolite.
^{b}7-Hydroxyfluphenazine.
^{c}Norclozapine or *N*-desmethylclozapine; possibly responsible for hematologic toxicity.
^{d}9-Hydroxyrisperidone (paliperidone); active moiety is risperidone plus 9-hydroxyrisperidone; 9-hydroxyrisperidone is equipotent with risperidone.

Based on Freudenreich O, Goff DC. Antipsychotics. In: Ciraulo DA, Shader RI, Greenblatt DJ, et al. eds. *Drug interactions in psychiatry.* 3rd ed. Philadelphia: Lippincott Williams & Wilkins, 2006:177–241.

KEY POINT

Note from Table 16.1 that most antipsychotics are metabolized by more than one enzyme or enzyme system. For example, haloperidol, olanzapine, and ziprasidone can be directly deactivated through CYP450-independent pathways. This serves as a built-in safety net, particularly if enzyme systems cannot be inhibited or induced, as is the case for aldehyde oxygenase.

It is useful to know that antipsychotics do not inhibit P450 enzymes (with the exception of 2D6, which is inhibited weakly by some antipsychotics) and that they do not induce P450 enzymes. In that respect, antipsychotics can be safely added to other treatment regimens.

It helps to recall a few general facts about the P450 system to anticipate drug interactions. First, some (but not all) isoenzymes can be induced or inhibited, the most important ones being 3A4 and 1A2. Antipsychotic drug levels will be lower in the presence of an inducer and higher in the presence of an inhibitor if either of these isoenzymes metabolizes the antipsychotic. The main inducer for 1A2 is not medication but smoking; consequently, smokers predictably require higher doses, compared to nonsmokers, of 1A2-dependent antipsychotics (i.e., olanzapine and clozapine). When smokers quit smoking, olanzapine and clozapine levels will rise and should be adjusted.

Second, some (but not all) enzymes show genetic polymorphism, the most important ones being 2D6. 2D6 shows genetic polymorphism, which results in four clinical phenotypes: so-called extensive (or normal) metabolizers, poor metabolizers (inactive enzyme), intermediate metabolizers (some enzyme activity), and ultrarapid metabolizers (greatly increased enzyme activity). There is no way of knowing your patient's 2D6 genotype without genotyping, although you can take into account a patient's ethnic background (e.g., some Middle Eastern and African populations have high rates of ultrarapid metabolizers) when considering side effects or nonresponse. With the advent of pharmacogenomics and personalized medicine, genechips are available for P450 genotyping. This seems to matter most for risperidone or older antipsychotics, which have significant 2D6-dependent metabolism: Ultrarapid metabolizers might never achieve plasma levels (and be accused of nonadherence), poor metabolizers will appear exquisitely sensitive to standard doses (extrapyramidal symptoms, or EPS).

 TIP

Undoubtedly, pharmacogenomics and personalized medicine will expand, and possibly one day we will be in a position to choose the dose and type of antipsychotic based on somebody's genetic makeup. In the interim, just check an antipsychotic drug level if you are unsure about the adequacy of the dosing. Antipsychotic drug levels can be obtained routinely for many antipsychotics.

CLINICAL APPROACH TO DRUG INTERACTIONS

You have two concerns with regard to drug interactions between antipsychotics and the other medicines your patient is taking: loss of antipsychotic efficacy and increased side effects. Usually, you only have to worry about loss of antipsychotic efficacy if a metabolic inducer is present (but realize that this could be an increase in smoking during times of stress). Pharmacodynamic interactions are rare and easy to anticipate (i.e., concomitant treatment with a dopamine agonist). Increased side effects are concerning if they lead to acute tolerability problems (e.g., akathisia or dystonic reactions), if they are life space, threatening (e.g., cardiac arrhythmias), or if they increase the long-term morbidity risk (e.g., for tardive dyskinesia or cardiovascular disease). Antipsychotics as a class have a very high margin of safety, and many patients tolerate even large increases in drug levels. For most antipsychotics, the risk from a higher drug level is EPS and sedation; for clozapine, however, it is seizures, and pimozide and mesoridazine/thioridazine become cardiotoxic.

 TIP

The most important safeguard against drug interaction, other than anticipation, is timely clinical follow-up. Ask your patient to call you or follow up with you in a week after you have added a medication or made a dose change. Record motor examination results and side-effect complaints prior to your change so that you have a baseline.

Before you add an antipsychotic (or any psychotropic) to your patient's regimen, consider the following points to avoid some problems related to drug interactions:

- Do not prescribe pimozide or mesoridazine/thioridazine unless under exceptional circumstances. Their cardiac safety profile does not justify the risk.
- Adjust antipsychotic dose based on smoking status (particularly for olanzapine and clozapine).
- Look at the overall medication regimen and, to anticipate problems, spot the main inducers or inhibitors from other specialties.
- Look at your patient and judge how the patient would tolerate a drug interaction: How sick is the patient medically? Frail patients might tolerate drug interactions very poorly.
- Consider antipsychotic drug levels in certain clinical situations (see next section).

 TIP

I have not found electronic drug-interaction databases helpful. In too many instances, drug interactions are based on theoretical interactions that in fact have never been described clinically or are so rare that they cannot guide your prescribing. Instead, I check PubMed by entering the two drugs and the search terms "pharmacokinetic" and "drug interaction." Many drug interactions are only a relative, not absolute, contraindication to combining medications.

Antipsychotic Drug Levels

Given the lack of dose–response curves for antipsychotics, it does not make sense to base dosing on antipsychotic drug levels, and it is not recommended routinely. However, antipsychotic drug levels can vary widely between patients for any given dose, and excluding the extremes of drug serum level (below detectable levels or dangerously high levels) can be important, particularly in complex clinical situations.

It is very useful to know that the elimination of antipsychotics follows linear pharmacokinetics: You need to measure a drug level only once during steady-state conditions to know the dose–serum level curve for this patient. Linear pharmacokinetics means: You double the dose, you double the level; you halve the dose, you halve the level.

CLINICAL VIGNETTE

A man in his 40s treated with carbamazepine 400 mg twice daily for epilepsy was on maintenance treatment with risperidone 3 mg twice daily for schizophrenia. When I first saw him, he was mildly paranoid. His risperidone serum level was nondetectable, and his risperidone metabolite level was 4 ng/nL (the lower end of therapeutic efficacy is around 10 ng/nL for the active moiety). His paranoia resolved after adjusting risperidone to 6 mg twice daily.

This is an example of an easily manageable and expectable drug interaction. I still find it useful to at least draw a serum drug level once to justify in my mind (and to insurance companies) the need for much higher than usual doses. Once you have established that the serum drug level is in fact subtherapeutic, you can adjust the dose based on clinical response.

DRUG INTERACTIONS BY MEDICATION CLASS

Antipsychotics with Antidepressants

The combination of antipsychotics with antidepressants is usually not problematic, but you need to follow your patients clinically as some antidepressants block metabolizing enzymes and lead to higher antipsychotic serum levels. Recall that there are clear differences between selective serotonin reuptake inhibitors (SSRIs) with regard to inhibiting P450 enzymes, and in complex situations you might want to choose an SSRI with few interactions (e.g., citalopram or venlafaxine). Fluoxetine is a strong inhibitor of 2D6, paroxetine of 3A4, and fluvoxamine of 1A2. Fluvoxamine should be avoided with clozapine and olanzapine as it can more than double serum levels of the antipsychotics.

Antipsychotics with Mood Stabilizers

This combination has a good safety record and is usually not problematic. Be careful, however, when you combine lithium with antipsychotics, since severe neurotoxic reactions (resembling a delirium and neuroleptic malignant syndrome) can occur. This combination can also lead to more EPS. Similarly, you often see more EPS, particularly tremor, in patients treated with valproate plus an antipsychotic. Valproate does not significantly interfere with the metabolism of antipsychotics. Carbamazepine is problematic in any medication regimen as it is a pan-inducer of P450 enzymes. As a rule of thumb, if you double the dose of the antipsychotic, you usually achieve sufficient plasma levels. I have had patients where I could not reach satisfactory drug levels (heroic doses can add substantial cost and might not be covered by the insurance company). In such cases, I would switch to oxcarbazepine, which has a lower (but not zero) propensity to induce 3A4. Lamotrigine can slightly increase some antipsychotic serum levels (via non-P450 mechanism) but the combination is clinically very well tolerated.

Antipsychotics with Benzodiazepines

The main concern here is pharmacodynamic in the form of additive central nervous system depression. There is a small literature of disastrous consequences (i.e., death) from giving benzodiazepine to clozapine patients. In clinical practice, carefully added benzodiazepines are well tolerated, and benzodiazepines are routinely used in patients on antipsychotics, including clozapine.

ADDITIONAL RESOURCES

Book

Freudenreich O, Goff DC. Antipsychotics. In: Ciraulo DA, Shader RI, Greenblatt DJ, et al. eds. *Drug interactions in psychiatry.* 3rd ed. Philadelphia: Lippincott Williams & Wilkins; 2006:177–241.—A chapter on antipsychotic drug interactions, which presents a more detailed and referenced version of this chapter.

Polypharmacy

Essential Concepts

- Polypharmacy is a fuzzy concept since, at the molecular level, antipsychotic monotherapy constitutes intrinsic polypharmacy.

- Appropriate reasons for combination treatments are as follows: added efficacy, supplemental symptom control, and adjunctive to increase tolerability.

- Fixing unnecessary polypharmacy requires patience and persistence, and can run counter to patient expectation.

- Time-limited trials and measuring outcomes are safeguards against polypharmacy. A small improvement in a symptom might be neither clinically meaningful nor justification of the long-term risk of the medication.

- Polypharmacy can flag treatment refractoriness.

- The acute treatment requires more and/or different medications than the maintenance phase (cf. oncology and cancer treatment).

- Hippocratic medicine demands that you treat diseases (and not simply symptoms) and that your intervention is effective (and not simply safe). Sometimes this would suggest doing nothing, one of the most difficult things to do in medicine.

"Simplify!"
—*Henry David Thoreau, American transcendentalist, 1817–1862*

Today, treatment with more than one medication is the norm, not the exception, for almost any disorder (e.g., hypertension, diabetes), including psychiatric disorders. Unless you have a framework that guides your prescribing practice, patients are at risk for unnecessary and harmful polypharmacy (and you are at risk of being quickly relegated to merely dispensing medications as the patient's "psychopharmacologist").

We have no agreed-upon definition of what constitutes "polypharmacy." In its narrowest sense, polypharmacy refers to the combination of two or more antipsychotics (same-class polypharmacy). In a slightly broader sense, polypharmacy refers to using two or more medications for the same condition. In its broadest sense, it is simple pill counting. Polypharmacy often has a negative connotation and implies the use of (too) many or unnecessary medications. What is rarely talked about is that at the molecular level, the concept might not be very meaningful at all (Freudenreich and Goff, 2003). Monotherapy with clozapine at the pill-counting level is polypharmacy at the molecular level—clozapine targets a multitude of receptors in the brain. With such a fuzzy concept, it is easy to see how one person's rational combination treatment becomes another person's irrational polypharmacy.

APPROPRIATE USE OF POLYPHARMACY

In medicine, "rational" polypharmacy is evidence of a good understanding of pathophysiology. Today, diabetes or hypertension is often treated with combinations that target different enzymes in the metabolic pathways or different receptors, acting synergistically. In schizophrenia, it is paradoxically the lack of knowledge of pathophysiology that justifies the empirical use of multiple medications. Polypharmacy is also logical for a complex disease like schizophrenia if you accept that antipsychotics are not "antischizophrenics": It makes sense to use other drug classes to target symptom clusters not ameliorated by antipsychotics.

These are then three reasonable clinical scenarios in which you would use more than one psychotropic (for details about which medications to combine, see Chapter 15 on ancillary medications):

- For added efficacy—If there is treatment resistance and you need to augment a partial response to your primary treatment.
- For supplemental symptom control—If you need to target specific symptoms, for example, insomnia or agitation not covered by your primary treatment.
- For treatment intolerance—If adjunctive medications are needed to improve tolerability of your primary treatment.

Although not a long-term strategy, engagement of patients with medications in a supportive mode can require the prescribing of medications with marginal or no benefit. This cannot be your principle mode of operation, and it is only justified if done safely. Nevertheless, some patients have learned that any complaint requires a medication. It will take time to unlearn such a counterproductive pattern, and you will have to teach your patients your philosophy of prescribing. In a patient who expects a medication, you will be perceived as empathic if you prescribe, and as punitive and withholding if you do not.

 TIP

It requires time and persistence to reverse a pattern of (unnecessary) polypharmacy in a patient. Note that both the act of giving *and withholding* medications has meaning for patients.

Treating patients who are only partially responsive to antipsychotics remains an art, and frequently a second antipsychotic is added despite a paucity of data (Freudenreich and Goff, 2002). Risperidone (Risperdal) augmentation of clozapine-treated patients is one example of an antipsychotic–antipsychotic combination that became prominent based on uncontrolled trials. Theoretically, adding dopamine blockade might be useful for some patients who need more dopamine blockade than the fairly loosely bound clozapine provides. Subsequent double-blind trials have not conclusively resolved the question of added efficacy for this particular combination, leaving the clinician with the need to decide on a case-by-case basis.

If you decide you must add a second antipsychotic (even though all schizophrenia guidelines recommend antipsychotic monotherapy), propose a time-limited trial, measure psychopathology, and judge if any change in psychopathology is clinically useful. If the change is not obvious to other people, it probably does not justify the added risks (Table 17.1).

TABLE 17.1. Risks of Antipsychotic Combination Treatment

Loss of "atypicality" of antipsychotics (if a first-generation antipsychotic is added to a second-generation antipsychotic)
Added toxicities (short and long term)
Expense
Drug interactions
Loss of efficacy

QUESTIONABLE POLYPHARMACY

"Just doing something" is a poor long-term strategy, particularly in the management of a lifelong disease. Not every complaint should make you reach for the prescription pad. Apart from cost, clear risks from polypharmacy are the potential for drug interactions, broadening side effects, or even limiting effectiveness if medication effects cancel each other out. The more medication, the more opportunity for patient mistakes.

 TIP

Polypharmacy can be a sign of poor treatment response. Make sure that each medication in a complex regimen is in fact useful (i.e., results in clinical improvement that justifies the risk of continuing it).

There are reasons other than true refractoriness, which are often not considered, that will lead to a patient accruing medications over time:

- Schizophrenia is treated according to an acute illness model with an expectation of complete resolution of symptoms and return to previous function (an often illusory goal).
- The benefit of the intervention is not measured (at a minimum, the effectiveness of the added medication for target symptoms should be measured). The benefit should extend beyond a mere change in a rating scale, but be clinically relevant.
- Unrecognized pseudo-refractoriness: For example, partial nonadherence or drug use are responsible for symptoms, not efficacy failure.
- Fear of worsening symptoms: The specter of "it could be worse" is raised in refractory patients who are very symptomatic despite maximum treatment, and because of this fear (and not because of proven benefit), no medication is ever discontinued.

Maintenance medications and those used during an acute illness phase are not necessarily the same. For example, induction chemotherapy for cancer is usually different from maintenance regimens. Similarly, the goals of psychiatric inpatient treatment (rapid stabilization and safety) are different from outpatient treatment (finding the best-tolerated mainte-nance regimen with the best long-term safety), requiring dif-ferent pharmacology.

CLINICAL VIGNETTE

Your patient with schizophrenia had been stable for many years on monotherapy with an antipsychotic while living in a group home, but becomes psychotic a few months after mov-ing into his own apartment. His old antipsychotic is restarted in the hospital since nonadherence is suspected as the main cause of his relapse. Because of the patient's level of agitation, valproate is added. When he does not seem to improve after 1 week, a second antipsychotic is added. Because he also complains about insomnia, an anxiolytic is added during the hospital stay as well. He is discharged on two antipsychotics, valproate, and an anxiolytic.

Unless you recognize that in this case medications were given for acute symptom control, patients like this are at risk for inappropriate long-term pharmacology, particularly if they are seen by different psychiatrists who do not know the longitudinal history (in this case, that the patient was rather well treated with antipsychotic monotherapy for many years). I have seen patients on ancient inpatient regimens that have simply been continued by each new psychiatrist that cared for the patient, in order not to "rock the boat."

HOW TO AVOID POLYPHARMACY— PHILOSOPHICAL THOUGHTS

The best protection against becoming a mere psychotropic pill pusher is having a conceptual view of the greater picture. There are two frameworks that I find useful in looking at my own medication prescribing. The first framework was most clearly articulated by my colleague (and former neighbor) Nassir Ghaemi: Do you practice Hippocratic medicine or not? Truly Hippocratic medicine is based on two principles, which Ghaemi (2006). summarizes as the Osler rule and the Holmes rule. Sir William Osler, the great physician, recog-nized that humans are all too willing to swallow an extra pill with the promise of a cure. He was a strong proponent of treating diseases, not symptoms (i.e., the Osler rule). Oliver Wendell Holmes, Sr. the admired physician and writer, challenged the unspoken assumption that drugs are potentially useful unless proven otherwise (in his days, the challenge was homeopathy) and suggested instead to consider drugs ineffective in the absence of evidence. His rule establishes the primacy of efficacy over safety when prescribing (i.e., the Holmes rule): You should not add a medicine simply because you think it is safe to do. Following these two rules makes you a true practitioner of Hippocratic medicine and lowers the risk of inappropriate polypharmacy. You either practice Hippocratic medicine or you practice symptom-based anti-Hippocratic medicine.

⬧ KEY POINT

You must treat schizophrenia-spectrum disorders as the syndromes that they are: For most patients, chronic illnesses for which you try to prevent relapse and improve function along the way. Without this longitudinal (and overarching view), any prescribing that is merely symptom-based will lead to polypharmacy since there is invariably another symptom to target. Sometimes, the most difficult thing is to do nothing.

In response to the Holmes rule in particular, it is often argued that lack of evidence does not suggest lack of efficacy. True, many clinical questions will never be studied in a clinical trial. (Cynics might say that once they are studied, they are often abandoned according to a well-known pattern of medical progress: Excitement from a small open-label trial, widespread penetration of a particular clinical practice, until it all ends with the publication of one or several negative double-blind, placebo-controlled trials that throw common practice into question.) However, available evidence for lack of efficacy is often conveniently ignored, and well-established treatments are forgone in favor of those with dubious claims.

A second framework I have found readily applicable was pointed out by the late psychiatrist Gerald Klerman. He suggested that most psychiatrists can put themselves in one of two camps: (a) hedonistic, or more willing to prescribe more, and (b) Calvinistic being more on the stingy side with psychotropics (Klerman, 1972). Just like you will not be liberal or conservative on all topics, you might find yourself to be more hedonistic with some patients (or some complaints) than with others. Give this distinction some thought the next time you ponder whether to prescribe or not to prescribe for a complaint of insomnia.

The anti-Hippocratic climate and hedonistic approach is of course not at odds with our cultural identity as a young and vigorous people. If suffering is seen as a disruption of a normal state of bliss, diseases are mere distractions and in need of a (preferably quick) fix. This becomes problematic if there is none. Without acknowledging this broader, sociocultural context and the expectations that this creates in your patient, you can find yourself fighting windmills when you try to practice Hippocratic medicine.

ADDITIONAL RESOURCES

Book

Ghaemi SN, ed. *Polypharmacy in psychiatry*. New York: Marcel Dekker; 2002.—The standard text on polypharmacy in psychiatry.

Article

Ghaemi SN. Hippocrates and Prozac: The controversy about antidepressants in bipolar disorder. *Primary Psychiatry.* 2006;13:51–58.—An excellent expose on the essence of Hippocratic medicine.

18 Psychologic Treatments— The Patient

Essential Concepts
- Supportive therapy is the pragmatic, real physician trying to help patients in the here-and-now with encouragement and advice. The foundation of supportive therapy is a good alliance with your patient.
- Cognitive–behavioral therapy (CBT) for psychosis is a promising ancillary treatment that tries to teach patients an alternative view of their symptoms and more effective coping strategies.
- Principles of CBT for psychosis can be easily integrated into treatment to address residual positive and negative symptoms not ameliorated by medications.
- Psychoeducation tries to improve how patients manage their disease by increasing knowledge.

> "A sense of a wider meaning to one's existence is what raises a man beyond mere getting and spending. If he lacks this sense, he is lost and miserable."
> —C. G. Jung (*Der Mensch und seine Symbole* (*MS 89*)/*Man and His Symbols*)

Simply dispensing antipsychotics, while treating the brain, does not treat the mind and soul of patients. In this chapter, I discuss supportive therapy, CBT, and psychoeducation as psychologic treatment modalities appropriate for most patients with schizophrenia. Psychoanalysis, or insight-oriented psychotherapies, when used alone is an inappropriate and woefully inadequate approach to treat schizophrenia, but you might see the occasional family still ask about psychoanalysis. That does not mean that in higher-functioning patients, elements from other therapies to address demoralization and existential suffering (the being thrown into this existence, Heidegger's *Geworfenheit*) should not be used. I have found elements from existential therapies (e.g., Victor Frankl's logotherapy) very applicable, but you might find other philosophies suit you more (see also Chapter 28, on depression and suicide, and the article on religion and spirituality in schizophrenia that is cited in the Additional Resources).

SUPPORTIVE THERAPY

"Supportive therapy" has a bad reputation, indicating that since nothing specific can be offered, one resorts to being merely supportive as opposed to attacking "root causes" in dynamic therapies. Apart from the questionable claim about the efficacy of many psychotherapies, at least for more severe disorders, supportive therapy is a useful treatment in its own right; in fact, most physicians in other specialties practice it all the time. Some might even argue that supportive therapy for patients with schizophrenia is one of the more demanding skills because of poor psychologic functioning of patients (e.g., those with primitive defense mechanisms).

I think of supportive therapy as a pragmatic encounter with the patient, focusing on today's problems ("*hic et nunc*— here and now") and how to solve them. If you want to get technical about supportive therapy, think of supportive therapy as the kind of therapy in which you benevolently use the good relationship (or positive transference) that you might have with your patient ("Yes, Doc, whatever you think is right for me"). It is rather difficult to be useful in the long run if your patient does not like you (which will happen). In supportive therapy, the topic of interest is not the transference or countertransference; be aware of, but do not interpret transferential issues. You know that you are doing something wrong if your patients leave the office more anxious than when they came in. You are a "real person." As the expert, you might not have all the answers, but recommendations and suggestions are helpful, too.

The talk in supportive therapy is conversational and natural. Avoid pauses. Talk about what you know: sports, family. To the uninitiated, this seems like chitchatting. In fact, you are doing a mental status examination, and you determine how much life the patient has other than being a professional patient. In patients you follow for many years, focusing only on areas of weakness and psychopathology is counterproductive. Focusing on areas of strength and pride (a patient might have great knowledge about baseball) serves the all-important purpose of fostering a good treatment alliance. A good alliance is the one thing that might save you when you have to make tough choices.

The use of medications is acceptable in supportive therapy and an important tool to decrease anxiety and other unpleasant affects.

Goals and Techniques of Supportive Therapy

You can look at three goals of supportive therapy:

- Ameliorate symptoms
- Decrease anxiety
- Enhance the triad of self-esteem, adaptive skill, and psychologic function (ego function)

These three goals define the boundaries with other therapies, in which personality change is the objective. In supportive psychotherapy, psychologic insight is not a primary goal and not seen as a prerequisite for change. Because psychologic change is not an objective (instead, increased adaptive function with what people have), shore up healthy defenses and do not challenge defenses.

Supportive techniques are direct and self-explanatory; you will use praise, encouragement, reassurance, and even advice and instruction. You will find yourself asking for clarification if patients are confusing in their utterances. Helping patients to rename experiences can subtly move patients to accept a different view of events.

CLINICAL VIGNETTE

Helga is a 45-year-old woman who has long-standing schizophrenia. She lives alone in an apartment a few houses away from her elderly mother, who was just in the hospital for an acute respiratory illness. You see Helga every other week when she comes for her clozapine clinic visit. Today, she is wearing new glasses.

One of the first things you might comment on is her new glasses. "I have not seen these glasses before, are they new?" The patient proudly affirms this, "Yes, I picked them out myself." In supportive therapy, it would be acceptable to praise the patient, "These look nice on you. You really picked well." This shows your approval and might enhance the patient's self-esteem. It would then be very appropriate to talk about the patient's mother. Saying "I heard your mother was in the hospital. How is she doing?" shows concern and helps with anxieties that the patient might have about her mother's illness. You could give direct advice: "How about going over to her house and cooking some soup for her?" If the patient describes insomnia related to worrying about her mother, adding a sedative to decrease anxiety and to help with sleep is appropriate (as opposed to focusing on the existential questions that the mother's illness might have provoked).

Simply being natural and stating the obvious (in this example, new glasses, concerns about mother's illness) is an essential ingredient in working with patients who suffer from schizophrenia.

COGNITIVE–BEHAVIORAL THERAPY

In recent years, CBT, originally developed as a treatment for depression, has developed some traction in the treatment of psychosis. Because the main impetus has come from research groups in Great Britain, it can be very difficult to find this treatment modality practiced in the United States. However, you can easily integrate some principles of CBT into routine clinical care.

CBT has several features that make it an attractive treatment modality. The reductionist and simplistic view of schizophrenia as a "brain disease" is rather pessimistic (and wrong) since it does not take into account the influence of environment and the relative frequency of psychotic symptoms in community samples. Van Os (2002) and others have argued strongly for a continuum model of psychosis. CBT tries to help patients develop a view of their disease that goes beyond a "broken brain" model of "madness," and, in doing so, broadens views of how symptoms come about and, what can be done about them. For example, normalization of psychotic experiences may reduce stigma.

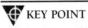 **KEY POINT**

CBT for schizophrenia makes several assumptions. For one, symptoms are conceptualized as the combined result of vulnerabilities (which could be biologic, social, or psychologic) and stressful life experiences. In this view, psychosis is seen as understandable and "normal." Symptoms are thought to be maintained by counterproductive appraisals and behaviors, which can be identified and changed. The CBT therapist identifies operative reasoning biases and challenges them through such techniques as cognitive restructuring or behavioral experiments. Examples of these biases include selective data gathering, jumping to conclusions, and overconfidence.

CBT is structured in a way that is very different from the usual clinic visit. Individual CBT sessions are usually held weekly, homework is assigned regularly, the CBT therapist adopts a directive (active) role, and sessions follow an agenda that is developed by both the patient and therapist at the beginning of each session. CBT sessions are designed to have a tone of collaborative discovery between the patient and therapist.

CBT is also time limited; once patients have completed a course of CBT (e.g., 16 to 20 sessions), they have learned a set of techniques to use, and it is then up to them to apply these techniques in the face of symptoms or difficult life situations. CBT is educational, and I have had patients tell me that it feels like being in school again.

Let me take delusions as a case in point to show how CBT can work. In a CBT framework, delusions are conceptualized as extreme beliefs that are held with a high level of conviction (but not necessarily always 100% conviction). This view opens delusions to Socratic questioning: "What makes you so sure? What is your evidence for this belief? Is it possible you are mistaken?" The CBT therapist aims to identify triggers of dysfunctional thoughts (using the ABC model, antecedent-belief-consequences, of CBT). After identifying cognitive biases (e.g., "all-or-nothing thinking"; "I am going to be attacked"), you can work on restructuring cognitions and changing maladaptive behaviors (e.g., leaving the subway in response to paranoia). You might set up a behavioral experiment, for example, having patients gradually increase the number of minutes they spend on the subway platform over the course of a week and recording whether they were attacked and what their associated anxiety ratings were. In the subway example, you would help patients identify and challenge automatic thoughts, and provide alternative explanations (e.g., a person might be looking at them on the subway platform because they appear nervous, rather than because the person is waiting to attack them).

Overall, the adaptation of CBT to treatment of psychosis is a very positive development. However, it is easy to oversell the benefit of CBT. Surgeons know very well that the most important predictor of outcome is patient selection, surgical candidate or not. CBT for psychosis can be useful for motivated patients who have some insight into the pathologic nature of their experiences and who are curious about them. In such patients, ancillary (to antipsychotics) CBT can be rather beneficial. Although CBT does not necessarily lead to symptom remission, patients who benefit are less stressed about their symptoms, perhaps because they have learned how to live with their symptoms better. I need to state clearly that for most patients CBT is no substitute for treatment with antipsychotics (which addresses the biologic vulnerability).

 TIP

Focus on function and goals, not symptoms, in patients who are hesitant to engage in symptom-based treatment. You want your patients to manage better and to achieve their goals, not necessarily to agree with you.

PSYCHOEDUCATION

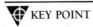 KEY POINT

Psychoeducation posits that increased knowledge about an illness leads to a better appreciation of the illness and its treatments, and thereby ultimately improved illness management. Patients should be experts in their illness and its management. Sometimes targeting the family for becoming illness experts yields more benefits (see next chapter).

Psychoeducation alone is insufficient since knowledge alone rarely leads to behavioral change. Nevertheless, psychoeducation has always been part of medicine and should be an integral part of any patient encounter, at least informally. Psychoeducation as a structured, curriculum-based activity with modules to learn about the illness is a fairly new idea in the mental health field. A possible model curriculum for schizophrenia should cover the illness and its treatments (symptoms, treatment, crisis management, recovery, and relapse), as well as wellness education (nutrition, healthy lifestyle, and exercise).

TIP

Many young patients use the Internet, which can replace "bibliotherapy" (a fancy term for learning by reading a book) to learn about schizophrenia and medications.

ADDITIONAL RESOURCES

Web Site

http://www.treatmentteam.com—This collaboration between a university and a drug company offers free materials for a model psychoeducation curriculum covering illness ("Team Solutions") and wellness ("Solutions for Wellness").

Books

Kingdon DG, Turkington D. *Cognitive therapy of schizophrenia.* New York: Guilford Press; 2005.—Practical summary of CBT for psychosis by British experts who helped shape the field. Pinsker H. *A primer of supportive psychotherapy.* Mahwah, NJ: Analytic Press; 1997.—First and still best book to explain supportive therapy.

Article

Mohr S, Brandt P-Y, Borras L, et al. Toward an integration of spirituality and religiousness into the psychosocial dimension of schizophrenia. *Am J Psychiatry.* 2006;163. 1952– 1959.—As I did not discuss the role of spirituality and religion for people with psychotic disorders, read this article as a good starting point.

19 Psychologic Treatments—
The Family

> **Essential Concepts**
> - Family members (often parents or siblings) can be the greatest resources your patient has. Help family members understand the illness, and let them help you take care of their child or sibling.
> - Families need more help when there is violence or the police are involved, or when there is frequent relapse or the need for reassurance is high.
> - Use the stress–diathesis model to explain the role of stressful environments (which can be the family environment) on the patient *without assigning blame*.

"Never tell people how to do things. Tell them what to do and they will surprise you with their ingenuity."
—*George S. Patton, US Army General, 1885–1945*

Schizophrenia affects everybody in the family. The dyadic view of patient and therapist is inappropriate and at times dangerous; you need eyes and ears in the community, and the family is your natural ally. Today, family work is more pragmatic and less theory driven than decades ago. In this chapter, I provide some suggestions on how to work with the family of your patient with schizophrenia, for everybody's benefit.

REASONS FOR FAMILY INVOLVEMENT

Families often play a crucial role in aiding treatment and recovery simply because most patients are still living with their families or have returned to the family home after a crisis or a hospitalization. Having a child or sibling with any illness is stressful for parents and siblings; having a child or sibling with psychosis is even more stressful. The concept of relational trauma might be useful: Even if family members do not suffer from overt symptoms, the illness nevertheless disrupts family function. In other areas of medicine, the burden on caregivers is openly acknowledged and addressed. Whereas family members who take care of patients with Alzheimer's disease are supported, families who have a member with schizophrenia all too often still suffer alone. Psychologically problematic is the fact that a child might be lost without being dead, leading to protracted grief that does not resolve.

Think of these as the goals of family involvement and interventions:

- Prevent family burnout to avoid abandonment of patients in the long run.
- Decrease isolation of families because of the stigma of mental illness.
- Alleviate guilt about having caused the illness.
- Provide realistic assessment of the illness and prognosis, not too positive, not too negative. Give hope that a good life is still possible.
- Teach families how to supervise medication adherence gently, without power struggles. Give the parent permission to be in charge of the medicine.
- Teach skills how to avoid and handle crises. Do this without being patronizing. Acknowledge the strengths that families have shown.
- Help reconnect patients with family members from whom they have been estranged, if this is desired.
- Reduce relapse rates by reducing stressful interactions among family members (see below, under Expressed Emotions).

Make it clear that you not only understand that families have concerns but that you value their involvement. A good working relationship with families goes a long way, as Tom Sawyer (and General Patton) recognized.

 TIP

Tom Sawyer understood how to motivate people to get a job done. Apply the Tom Sawyer approach to problem solving: Identify what needs to be done, then delegate appropriately (i.e., know the limits of family responsibilities). There is no reason that a family member cannot try to get a discharge summary from a hospitalization that happened in Alaska. (I found the Tom Sawyer approach mentioned in Kanter, 1996.)

As important as it is to help families help their sick relative, you also need to help patients deal with their families. While I always talk with family members who have accompanied a patient to the appointment, I also always talk to the patient alone as well to address concerns that the patient has about his or her family.

SELECTION OF FAMILIES

All families that want to be involved in the treatment of their child or sibling should be involved in it, but the degree and type of involvement vary. For many families, you simply being available for questions by phone or e-mail is sufficient. Even in those "low-maintenance cases," I ask all my patients to bring one family member to one of the appointments "to touch base" at least once a year.

 TIP

Know who is in the patient's family. I have found that it works best if you set aside a visit during which you literally draw a family tree with the patient. I do this even with patients I have known for years: "Let me go over your family today in a little more detail." Figure out, "Who lives where? When was the last time you saw your brother? What is your father doing?"

There are two situations in which it is mandatory to work more extensively with families: first-episode patients and problematic families. Family work may be especially important during the first episode, as relatives tend to experience the greatest amount of distress during the first 2 years of illness. The eminent British cross-cultural psychiatrist Julian Leff has identified several red flags for families who need more help than just education (Table 19.1).

TABLE 19.1. Red Flags for Intensive Family Involvement

- Frequent arguments that lead to violence
- Families who call 911
- Adherent patients who relapse more than once per year
- Relatives with frequent staff contact for reassurance

WORKING WITH FAMILIES

The first step is to help family members understand what schizophrenia is (and what it is not). You cannot expect the average person to know the difference between schizophrenia, "split personalities," or sociopathy. Without education, grossly distorted "personalized lay views" result.

Most family members want to know how they can best help, including what not to do. A useful model to discuss the interaction of genes and environment is the stress–diathesis model, which I prefer over the expressed emotions model (see Expressed Emotions, below).

⚙ KEY POINT

It helps to explain schizophrenia as a disorder that leaves the sufferer very sensitive to the environment, including the family situation (stress–diathesis model). Medications buffer against social stress to some extent, but sometimes the environment (i.e., the family atmosphere) needs to be changed as well. In that way, families can positively affect how well somebody is doing. This does not mean that families are to blame if patients are not doing well; there can be many reasons for this.

Here is a list of very concrete steps to help the family of somebody with schizophrenia:

- Refer families to the National Alliance on Mental Illness (NAMI) for support in their community (see Additional Resources). NAMI is the largest and oldest grassroots organization dedicated to helping families who have a relative with mental illness, particularly schizophrenia. There are chapters in all 50 states.
- Many NAMI chapters offer psychoeducation for families via a family-taught course, "Family-to-Family."
- Provide reading suggestions to learn about schizophrenia (see Additional Resources).
- Help develop skills for crisis intervention (and how to avoid crises), and an explicit crisis plan. Prescribe new solutions for recurrent problems.
- Be available. Do not hide behind regulatory barriers.
- Involve family from the get-go and keep them involved.

- Set a tone that makes families allies. Never blame (i.e., think twice before you make a statement that contains "should" or "shouldn't").

If available, so-called multiple family groups in which several families are seen together can offer advantages; this group format might provide some corrective: "Some families are worse off. My problems are not unique." Do not forget that while you have seen hundreds of cases of schizophrenia, families have seen one. Families might give each other helpful suggestions about local resources and strategies as well.

 TIP

At some point, let the family identify one family member who will communicate with you and whom you can contact with urgent matters. Ask other members of the family to funnel concerns through that "family spokesperson."

Expressed Emotions

No section on family treatment would be complete without mentioning the concept of expressed emotions (EE). The EE construct was based on the clinical observation that some patients relapsed more rapidly than others following hospital discharge, depending on the environment they returned to. Those who returned to their families had higher relapse rates than those with different dispositions. Subsequent studies have confirmed that some families, so-called high-EE families, create a stressful family atmosphere that doubles the relapse rate compared to low-EE families. High-EE families are characterized by three key factors: frequent criticism, hostility, and overinvolvement (Heru, 2006).

High EE in and of itself is not pathologic; many families have a high-EE style. Some families might be naturally more laid back toward psychotic behavior. Conversely, I would not underestimate the toll on any healthy family that has to cope with an ill relative who might not only not get substantially better but who in addition seems to be sabotaging treatment—by not taking medication, for example. Although families cannot be blamed for being high EE, the atmosphere in such families can be very stressful for somebody with schizophrenia (or such other disorders as depression).

⊕ KEY POINT

For some patients with schizophrenia, family atmosphere matters and can contribute to a psychotic relapse. Critical relatives who hold patients responsible for their illness seem to have the most impact on potential relapse. Find out from the patient, "On a scale from 1 to 10, how critical is your family of you?," and gently address this with the family.

The overinvolvement seen in some families is often entrenched and the result of severe disability on the part of the patient. I have seen patients who are shepherded around every minute of the day. While counterintuitive, prescribing reduced contact with the ill family member is sometimes necessary since patients need time to themselves to grow up and develop some degree of independence. This could be as simple as letting the patient go to the movies alone.

CLINICAL VIGNETTE

After developing psychosis in his second year of college and following a psychiatric hospitalization, Alexander finds himself living at home again with his parents. He has responded well to the antipsychotic and is waiting for a community college class to start. He sleeps in and stays up late (but sleeps only 8 hours total). He denies feeling fatigued from the medications. His mother is constantly berating him for not getting up and "doing something." She wants his medications to be changed, "so he is more motivated."

This is an example of a fairly common scenario that creates stress for everybody and that can be reduced with some gentle education: A delayed sleep–wake cycle (i.e., "sleeping in") is physiologically normal for younger people, getting up at 7 A.M. bright-eyed and bushy-tailed is unusual, particularly if there is no reason to do so. I explain to patients and families that "it is twice as difficult for somebody with a mental illness to look half as normal," to teach them the importance of not pathologizing every observation. Even if getting up late were a sign of negative symptoms, creating stress for the patient is counterproductive. You could prescribe no contact before noon.

ADDITIONAL RESOURCES

Web Sites

http://www.nami.org—The Web site of the National Alliance on Mental Illness, which has chapters in all 50 states. Family members can get education and support through their local chapter.

Books

Karp DA. *The burden of sympathy: How families cope with mental illness.* New York: Oxford University Press; 2001.—A sociologist brings to life the vicissitudes of caring for a mentally ill family member in postmodern America. A required reading for families and psychiatrists.

Mueser KT, Gingerich S. *The complete family guide to schizophrenia: Helping your loved one to get the most out of life.* New York: Guilford Press; 2006.—A new, eminently practical guide for families about how best to help their relative with schizophrenia.

Torrey EF. *Surviving schizophrenia.* 5th ed. New York: Harper-Collins; 2006.—The standard guide for families by one of the leaders in the field of psychiatry; now in its fifth edition.

20 Psychiatric Rehabilitation

Essential Concepts

- Psychiatric rehabilitation and psychiatric treatment are separate, yet equally important, complementary components of schizophrenia care.
- Psychiatric rehabilitation focuses on function and role outcomes, not on symptoms. A new rehabilitation focus is wellness.
- A rehabilitation assessment clarifies the patient's goals and then assesses skills and supports needed to attain these goals.
- Work adds so much to our self that vocational rehabilitation should be given utmost attention, even though the odds for competitive employment for patients with schizophrenia are less than 1 in 5.

"There can be no transforming of darkness into light and of apathy into movement without emotion."
—C. G. Jung 1875–1961, Swiss psychiatrist

It requires more than medicines to treat schizophrenia. For optimal results, orthopedic surgery is followed by rehabilitation in the form of physical therapy (PT). Similarly, psychiatric treatment (i.e., pharmacologic and psychologic treatments) needs to be accompanied by psychiatric or psychosocial rehabilitation. Psychiatric treatment and psychiatric rehabilitation are not mutually exclusive but rather complement each other. I will follow the tradition in the mental health field and juxtapose psychiatric treatment with rehabilitation even though you could consider rehabilitation to be one of the tools of treatment at your disposal. Psychiatric rehabilitation has a strong tradition of de-emphasizing professional involvement, probably rooted in the times when many patients were simply warehoused in "rehabilitation units." When you read the rehabilitation literature, you will note that patients are often called "clients" or "consumers" in an effort to empower patients by de-emphasizing the traditional power differential between physicians and patients. You will further notice that rehabilitation services usually embrace a "recovery-oriented philosophy," with hope being a fundamental ingredient in rehabilitation, and an emphasis on function and strengths, not dysfunction and weakness.

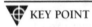 KEY POINT

One useful definition of "psychosocial rehabilitation" is the following by Bachrach: "A therapeutic approach that encourages a mentally ill person to develop his or her fullest capacities through learning and environmental supports." This definition acknowledges the need for patient participation as well as the need for environmental adjustments.

Rehabilitation starts as early as possible and is not contingent on symptom resolution, which can be elusive. However, it is difficult to fully participate in rehabilitation programs if you are too ill. This is similar to pain and PT: Your ability to participate in PT is limited if you are in too much pain, but very possible with some modicum of pain control.

REHABILITATION GOALS

Psychiatric rehabilitation does not focus on symptoms but on role outcomes. To avoid the inflation of the term rehabilitation to include any program that the patient attends, a pioneer of rehabilitation in the United States, William Anthony, has suggested considering skill building to be the critical element of rehabilitation. If an activity does not involve skill building, it is better called enrichment. Going bowling with peers is enrichment, not rehabilitation in this narrow sense (unless the goal is to build the skill of becoming a proficient bowler). In a broader sense, however, even bowling can be rehabilitation if a stated goal is teaching social skills and not merely killing time. Good programs focus on acquiring one specific skill at a time and provide ongoing support down the road, as needed. Successful rehabilitation decreases social isolation, improves skills and confidence, enlarges social networks, and increases the chances of returning to work or school. Successful rehabilitation should allow the patient to be a member of society and contribute to the greatest extent possible. Psychiatric rehabilitation is complicated by a sociocultural context of stigma, exclusion, and discrimination. Changing societal attitudes and discriminatory laws are part of rehabilitation in a larger sense.

The starting point for rehabilitation is helping patients figure out or clarify their goals and then provide them with the skills and supports they need to attain these goals. It should be obvious that rehabilitation must be tailored to the individual patient's needs and abilities.

 TIP

A good rehabilitation question to ask: "Where would you like to be 1 year from now?" Based on the answer (e.g., get GED), you need to figure the skills required to get there (e.g., take GED classes) and the supports needed (e.g., where to enroll a patient, financial supports, individual tutors).

It will come as no surprise that most patients have dreams and aspirations similar to the rest of us: To live a life with security, friends, a sense of belonging, and with something meaningful to do. "Wellness" is a new focus of rehabilitation. Not all patient goals are psychiatric rehabilitation goals in its narrow sense (skill building). Instead, patients often have a host of social needs that are nondisease issues, for example, poverty or homelessness that must be dealt with before educational or vocational rehabilitation attempts. It is difficult to learn a skill if you are hungry and have no place to sleep. Note that "housing" is not a psychiatric rehabilitation goal per se, even though stable and secure housing is obviously desired and necessary for rehabilitation. There is an advantage of restricting rehabilitation to skill building as you can design programs that address needed skills and provide support: Maintaining housing can be easily conceptualized as a rehabilitation goal if loss of housing is the result of poor budgeting skills resulting in eviction because of not paying rent. What rehabilitation can do is provide supported housing and teach budgeting skills.

Competitive employment in some capacity would be a crucial rehabilitation achievement that unfortunately is rarely achieved in our society if you have schizophrenia. Work defines us and gives us meaning, beyond the mundane consideration of allowing us to buy things. Unfortunately, in the United States less than 15% of patients with schizophrenia in the Clinical Antipsychotic Trials of Intervention Effectiveness (CATIE) cohort worked competitively (Rosenheck et al., 2006). True, not everybody wants to work, not everybody can work, and working does not make sense for everybody economically. However, the reasons for this poor functional outcome might go deeper and can leave us with some pessimism. The sociologist Sennett has used the term "specter of uselessness" to indicate a dilemma in a society built on modern meritocracy in which new values are no longer skills but adaptability, and employees are judged by potential and not by actual skills and achievements. These larger, socioeconomic factors that lead to lack of opportunity are huge impediments to rehabilitation.

It would be foolish to focus merely on strengths and lose sight of real-world impairment and deficits. Psychiatrists can be very useful in delineating cognitive impairment (e.g., by ordering neuropsychologic testing) and help pace and prioritize rehabilitation efforts. While I am not opposed to adopting the more positive language of rehabilitation when appropriate, I suggest a healthy sense of realism and frank discussion of impairments and impediments to rehabilitation as well. Motivational impairment is one of the biggest obstacles to successful psychiatric rehabilitation that is often not acknowledged enough.

CLINICAL VIGNETTE

Andreas is a 45-year-old man with deficit schizophrenia. He lives in a group home with other patients who also have schizophrenia. Every morning the "program van" comes and picks up the patient and the other group home members to go to the "recovery-oriented" (from the program brochure) psychosocial day program where he spends 5 hours every workday either in groups or in a common area. Staff members have signed him up for the groups that he must sit through. In the offered groups, he sits and waits until time is up. Sometimes he protests that he would rather stay in the group home; this is usually ignored.

This patient represents a not so rare but rarely talked about problem: You cannot rehabilitate *to* people, only *with* them. While rehabilitation goals will be determined by motivated persons, what about those who are content sitting at home doing nothing? Does family opinion or staff opinion matter, or are rehabilitation goals solely determined by patients? I am not proposing that there is an easy answer, but simply pointing out that forcing program participation is closer to social control than rehabilitation. At a minimum, for any program that you send your patient to, ask yourself what the goals of the programs are and if you would send a family member to the program.

Providing false hope by setting unrealistic and unattainable goals with resulting failure is a poor prescription. Nevertheless, have flexibility in setting goals and humility about your ability to predict the future; I have been proved wrong both ways: Some patients will surprise you with talents and accomplishments that seemed impossible; others will do poorly. In all cases, I remain hopeful for small improvements with time.

REHABILITATION TOOLS

Psychosocial rehabilitation requires a wide range of services (Table 20.1). The best services also serve real-world patients, not the ideal patient. For example, integrated substance use programs accept patients who have schizophrenia and a substance use disorder instead of splitting services between two different programs with different program philosophies. Ideally, psychosocial rehabilitation programs are a step toward independence and attendance is not an end in itself.

TABLE 20.1. Psychiatric Rehabilitation Tools for Schizophrenia

Modality	Goals
Social skills training	Improve social adjustment and independent living skills
Supported vocational rehabilitation	Return to competitive, paid employment
Supported employment	Enhance work tenure
Supported housing	Enhance community tenure and prevent homelessness
Assertive community treatment	Reduce psychiatric hospitalizations and risk to community
Case management	Coordinate rehabilitation and treatment services
Entitlement programs	Satisfy basic needs so patient is able to participate in rehabilitation

One well-known and successful rehabilitation program is the clubhouse model that was started in the 1950s by patients themselves after they were discharged from state hospitals as part of deinstitutionalization. There are now clubhouses in many major cities in the United States and other countries. Clubhouses engage patients by simply allowing them to be part of something normal. Once members are ready, they participate in running the program and learn new skills (e.g., cooking, budgeting). The clubhouse model takes its strengths from the strengths of peer support.

Many so-called rehabilitation programs are not rehabilitation programs in the skill-building sense. Many are mostly social programs with recreational activities. I do not want to minimize the importance of such programs for individual patients, as they might provide them with the only socially meaningful opportunity they have. Some patients are in fact not ready for rehabilitation, and such programs (also known as drop-in centers) provide the basis for engagement as a limited yet necessary first goal. However, from a larger perspective, creating psychiatric ghettos where patients live in parallel to "real" life cannot be rehabilitation and is problematic.

The way services are delivered is important because it has to be tailored to the patient's needs. Office-based case management for patients who can work with a case manager or assertive community treatment for patients who need to be seen in the home are examples of how to organize services so patients get the support they need.

Welfare programs that are based on needs alone include Supplemental Security Income (SSI); Medicaid; and special vouchers for housing, transportation, or food stamps (Table 20.2). Social Security Disability Insurance (SSDI) is different in that it can provide income to people who have worked and paid Social Security taxes before becoming disabled. Medicare similarly is an entitlement based on previous contributions. Note again that payments from any of these programs are tools for rehabilitation, and "getting SSI" does not constitute "rehabilitation." It is often worthwhile to apply for SSI or SSDI since eligibility will qualify patients for other assistance programs (e.g., Medicaid or state rehabilitation programs).

Rehabilitation requires that you work as part of an interdisciplinary team of which many team members might have philosophical views different from yours. Many team members you will never meet; some team members will have great titles but accomplish very little for your patients. You need to figure out who can do what for you and the patient.

TABLE 20.2. Entitlement and Welfare Programs

SSI	Federal assistance for the aged, blind, or disabled, based on financial need alone
SSDI	Federal insurance benefit based on previous work and payment of Social Security taxes
Medicaid	Federal health insurance program for low-income people administered by the state (with different rules for eligibility in different states); known by different names in some states for example, in Massachusetts, the program is known as MassHealth
Medicare	Federal health insurance program for people over 65 and other groups

 TIP

Make a list of services and organizations involved in the patient's rehabilitation. Consider yourself as the (at least informal) leader of an invisible team. Delegate, but avoid wishful thinking: The night-shift person in the group home you are dealing with might have little understanding of schizophrenia and should not be burdened with tasks beyond his or her expertise

ADDITIONAL RESOURCES

Web Sites

http://www.iccd.org—The International Center for Clubhouse Development; provides information and listings by state of certified clubhouses modeled after the first one, Fountain House in New York City.

IV

PROGNOSTIC CONSIDERATIONS FOR PSYCHOTIC DISORDERS

21

Medical Morbidity and Mortality

Essential Concepts

- Physical health and wellness matter as much as mental health to patients with schizophrenia. Reducing premature deaths from cardiac disease is an important treatment goal.
- Routine health monitoring in conjunction with primary care to prevent medical morbidity and mortality should be implemented. This includes preventive health care (e.g., eye examinations colonoscopy), vaccinations (e.g., influenza), and screening for infectious diseases (e.g., human immunodeficiency virus [HIV], hepatitis).
- Seven of ten patients with schizophrenia smoke. To reduce cardiovascular mortality and lung diseases, help patients quit.
- Four of ten patients with schizophrenia have the metabolic syndrome. Preventing weight gain and the metabolic syndrome are important to reduce cardiac mortality. Weight control requires lifestyle modification.
- Switching antipsychotics for metabolic reasons is a decision that must take into account the risk of psychiatric instability.

"Mens sana in corpore sano."
"A sound mind in a sound body."
Juvenal, Roman poet, late 1st and early 2nd century

It has been estimated that having schizophrenia shortens average life expectancy by at least 15 years. Although some of the excess mortality comes from suicide, cardiovascular disease has emerged as the most important cause of premature death. In the Clinical Antipsychotic Trials of Intervention Effectiveness (CATIE), patients had a fourfold increased 10-year cardiac risk over the general population, with higher rates of several major cardiac risk factors (smoking, diabetes, hypertension, and low high-density lipoprotein, or HDL) (Goff et al., 2005a). Consequently, the role of the psychiatrist can no longer be simply to keep patients out of psychiatric hospitals. Instead, addressing modifiable cardiovascular disease risk factors, particularly smoking and obesity (with its associated metabolic syndrome), have become an important aspect of psychiatric care for patients with schizophrenia. With poor physical health, your patient might die mentally well, but at an early age (the proverbial operation that was a success but the patient died).

Focusing on physical health early, when patients start taking medications, might prevent some of the morbidity that we see in today's cohort of middle-aged patients.

 TIP

Calculate each patient's 10-year Framingham cardiac risk (see Additional Resources). An increased risk might motivate some patients to quit smoking and change their lifestyle.

ROUTINE HEALTH MONITORING

Concern yourself with the physical health of your patients. As a psychiatrist, you often have much more contact with a psychiatric patient than does the primary care physician (PCP), and you might be in a much better position to monitor physical health and to advise behavioral changes. I suggest that you assume primary responsible for at least two aspects of physical health: smoking cessation and monitoring the effects of the medications that you prescribe, especially weight gain and metabolic problems.

Record the following medical information in every patient chart:

- Smoking status as a "vital sign" (e.g., 1 pack per day); note nicotine dependence, if present.
- Body mass index (BMI), not just weight; note if overweight or obese.
- Dyslipidemia, diabetes, or hypertension, if present (See WELL CARD Dyslipidemia, Hyperglycemia, Hypertension in Appendix C).
- Metabolic syndrome, if present (see WELL CARD Metabolic Syndrome in Appendix C).
- Activity level (e.g., inactive, walks, exercises three times a week).

If you detect a medical problem, you can treat what you are comfortable with or defer to a PCP. Even if your patient has a PCP, there is no harm in reinforcing the need for preventive screening (e.g., eye examinations or colonoscopy), reviewing vaccination requirements (e.g., influenza vaccine in the fall), or suggesting testing for infectious diseases when indicated (e.g., tuberculosis, hepatitis C virus, HIV). Your patients might trust your advice more than you realize, and your intervention might actually lead to their accessing some preventive health care.

 TIP

PCP offices are a resource to you, not a burden: Work with them. Make a phone call, e-mail, or write a note to introduce yourself. PCPs are often pleasantly surprised if a psychiatrist takes an interest in the physical health of their patients.

SMOKING

Smoking is one of the most important modifiable risk factors for cardiac disease. This is such an important topic that I have dedicated an entire chapter to it (Chapter 24).

 KEY POINT

See smoking as the threat it is to your patients, both in terms of health risk and as a potential financial hardship (i.e., patients can spend more than one third of their income on cigarettes). Psychiatrists, given their expertise in addictions and their frequent visits with patients relative to primary care, are ideally positioned to take the lead in smoking cessation.

WEIGHT GAIN AND OBESITY

Helping patients maintain a healthy weight or lose excess weight is probably the most vexing and maddening medical problem that you will try to address. The importance of preventing weight gain or promoting weight loss lies in preventing the medical consequences of being overweight or obese, including the metabolic syndrome. The metabolic syndrome is a constellation of factors that increase the risk for heart disease. Obesity has a host of other complications that adversely affect quality of life (e.g., daytime sedation from obstructive sleep apnea).

 TIP

Calculate each patient's BMI and put in your note (see WELL CARD Body Mass Index in Appendix C). You will be surprised how many patients for whom you did not suspect a weight problem are overweight or obese according to their BMI. Also determine for each patient if they suffer from the metabolic syndrome (see WELL CARD Metabolic Syndrome in Appendix C).

Clinical Management

A cynic might say that we have no treatment to prevent weight gain—the rates of obesity in the United States keep increasing every year in every state, despite billions spent on "healthier" foods and weight loss drugs. You are now trying to prevent weight gain against this background of an ever-increasing BMI in the general population; and you are attempting this in a population that might be less motivated. To add insult to injury, our medications clearly exacerbate any such weight gain that might occur naturally. I find it useful to view psychotropics as one more risk factor toward weight gain that patients must take into account (as opposed to attributing all and any weight gain to medications alone). Obviously, you would prefer to choose an antipsychotic with the least liability toward weight gain to prevent added iatrogenic morbidity. Suffice it to say that this is not always possible: Our most effective antipsychotics, olanzapine and clozapine, are also the most problematic ones with regard to weight gain.

KEY POINT

As antipsychotic-induced weight gain and metabolic problems often come together, monitor them together when you start an antipsychotic:

Get baseline weight, height, and waist circumference
Get baseline fasting glucose and fasting lipid profile
Get baseline blood pressure

Check weight every visit for 6 months, then quarterly
Recheck fasting glucose and fasting lipid profile after 3 months, then yearly
Recheck blood pressure after 3 months, 6 months, and then yearly

More stringent monitoring can be clinically necessary. However, perfect is the enemy of good: Start monitoring now and do your best to implement some longitudinal monitoring. Most importantly, recognize early weight gain and intervene early (consider a 5% weight gain significant). (See WELL CARD Physical Health Monitoring in Schizophrenia in Appendix C for a tabulated scheme.)

Without therapeutic lifestyle changes (TLC), the new term for exercise and diet, it will be very difficult to treat obesity meaningfully. While you want to be an advocate for healthy living, guard against becoming a crusader for better-than-well (Fitzgerald, 1994). Patients should not lose weight to please you. You cannot give them the impression that failure to lose weight is a personal insult to you and causes you to be disappointed in them. Weight loss in and of itself is also not the goal; healthier living and increasing fitness is. Thus, do not focus on simply how much weight was lost but how the efforts of better eating and of more walking are beneficial.

For all patients, have realistic, long-term weight goals. I would encourage the following four behavioral changes that would have a positive effect in the long term, if implemented.

- Normal portions for whatever is eaten. Teach patients about portion sizes so they appreciate how much they consume. Do not micromanage what they eat.
- Have patients weigh themselves every week to catch small but steady weight gain.
- No desserts. (As a compromise for New England, limit donuts to once a week for breakfast).
- No soft drinks, water instead.

 TIP

Get your patient to be more active. Stress the benefits of an active lifestyle to the patient Regular exercise *even in the absence of weight loss* can improve the metabolic syndrome. Always be reasonable: How likely is it that a person who never ran a mile will start jogging regularly? Perhaps the person used to swim and can join the local YMCA again. Perhaps taking the stairs instead of the elevator can be literally the first step.

The role of weight loss medications for antipsychotic-induced weight gain is unclear. Effective short-term treatments exist but are not without risks. For example, in a 12-week trial, patients with olanzapine-associated weight gain lost 8.3 lb when given sibutramine, compared to 2.4 lb in placebo-treated patients, albeit at the cost of a slight increase in systolic blood pressure (Henderson et al., 2005b). Selected patients might benefit from time-limited trials of available weight loss medications (e.g., sibutramine) or other remedies that have been found effective in small trials (e.g., amantadine). If weight loss is insignificant after 6 months or so on one of those medications, you can always stop the trial. Even seemingly small decreases in body weight might have beneficial effects, however, on metabolic parameters. Suffice it to say that in an ideal world weight loss medications are to be combined with behavioral interventions, although desperate situations require desperate measures. The prevention or reversal of antipsychotic-induced weight gain and metabolic problems is an active area of research (e.g., by adding metformin to the antipsychotic).

Overweight patients often request a change in their antipsychotic to one with less weight-gain liability. This can be a reasonable strategy (and might be more effective than trying to lose weight with exercise or by adding weight loss medications), and the effect of switching overweight patients with hypercholesterolemia to aripiprazole is currently being studied in a large National Institute of Mental Health (NIMH) trial, Comparison of Antipsychotics for Metabolic Problems (CAMP).

⦿ KEY POINT

In many cases you will have to weigh the risks and benefits of switching from a stable antipsychotic regimen to a generally less weight-inducing antipsychotic, ziprasidone or aripiprazole. This is an important clinical decision that you have to make with the patient (and family members). Do not sacrifice psychiatric stability on the altar of weight loss.

ADDITIONAL RESOURCES

Web Sites

http://www.cdc.gov/nip—The Centers for Disease Control National Immunization Program, with guidelines for adult vaccinations.

http://epss.ahrq.gov/ePSS/index.jsp—This site from the US Department of Health and Human Services allows you so search for screening recommendations based on a patient's age and sex.

http://hp2010.nhlbihin.net/atpiii/calculator.asp—A tool to calculate your 10-year cardiac risk (for myocardial infarction or death in the next 10 years) based on the Framingham cardiac risk factors (age, gender, smoker, total cholesterol, HDL cholesterol, and systolic blood pressure); note that the risk calculation assumes you do not have diabetes.

http://www.healthierus.gov/dietaryguidelines—From the US Department of Agriculture and the Department of Health and Human Services for those who want to get serious about improving their diet; many links (e.g., to the food pyramid).

Articles

Fitzgerald FT. The tyranny of health. *N Engl J Med.* 1994;331: 196–198.—Mandatory reading so you do not become a health zealot.

Marder SR, Essock SM, Miller AL, et al. Physical health monitoring of patients with schizophrenia. *Am J Psychiatry.* 2004; 161:1334– 1349.—Important consensus guidelines on health monitoring.

Goff DC, Cather C, Evins AE, et al. Medical morbidity and mortality in schizophrenia: Guidelines for psychiatrists. *J Clin Psychiatry.* 2005;66:183–194.—Health monitoring guidelines from the Massachusetts General Hospital (MGH) Schizophrenia Program.

HIV/AIDS and Serious Mental Illness

Essential Concepts

- Patients with schizophrenia are at increased risk for HIV infection.
- The Centers for Disease Control and Prevention (CDC) recommends screening for HIV as part of routine medical care (i.e., regardless of risk factors): Screen your patients with schizophrenia for HIV.
- Have a candid discussion of HIV risk factors: Drug use and sexual practices. It is a myth that patients with schizophrenia are asexual.
- Help patients reduce their risk for contracting or transmitting HIV by educating them about HIV, tailored to their understanding.
- Identify and treat psychiatric obstacles to antiretroviral therapy (ART) adherence (in particular depression, active substance use (cocaine and alcohol), uncontrolled psychosis).
- Take drug interactions and HIV disease stage into account when choosing and dosing antipsychotics.

"The biggest disease today is not leprosy or tuberculosis, but rather the feeling of being unwanted."
—Mother Teresa of Calcutta, **Noble** Peace Prize 1979

As a group, patients with so-called severe and persistent mental illness (SPMI), which includes schizophrenia, are at higher risk for HIV/AIDS than the general population. Exact numbers are hard to come by since seroprevalence of HIV infection is often based on highly selected samples of convenience done in epicenters of the HIV epidemic. In a cohort of 320 first admissions for psychosis in all of Suffolk County, NY (also known epidemiologically as "semirural Long Island"), 3.8% of patients were known to have HIV/AIDS. This 3.8% is an estimate of the *minimum* prevalence since the cohort was not systematically tested for HIV. The main cause of death in this cohort of young people was AIDS!

 TIP

The CDC recommends opt-out screening* for HIV as part of regular medical care in all health care settings (Branson et al., 2006). Screening is no longer based on risk factors. Thus, offer HIV screening to every patient with schizophrenia that you treat, *regardless of risk*. You are often in the best position to get this done. Consider screening for hepatitis C as well.

One obvious risk factor for HIV infection is current or past injection drug use. However, sexual transmission is the most common mode of infection for patients with schizophrenia. This is sometimes not suspected because providers consider their patients asexual, an assumption that is simply wrong. In one study of 95 patients with schizophrenia who were interviewed face-to-face about their sexual activity, about half had been sexually active in the previous 6 months (Cournos and Guido, 1994). What is problematic is that sexual encounters are often unplanned and might occur with populations at risk for sexually transmitted diseases. Add to this poor judgment and lack of social competence in negotiating sexual encounters, and many patients will have a sexual encounter in which no condoms are used. I think many patients are simply taken advantage of. In some cases, trading sex for money or drugs is a patient's reality. Although many patients have reasonable knowledge of HIV, this is certainly not true of all patients, and misinformation about HIV is frequent in more severely ill patients. Remember also that knowledge does not necessarily change behaviors.

The treatment of patients with both schizophrenia and HIV is complicated by several factors:

- Cognitive impairment, which requires modification of the usual HIV education. Repeated role playing and concrete practice may be necessary.
- Drug interactions; consider the antipsychotic serum drug level.

*Currently, opt-out screening conflicts with most state laws. In Massachusetts for example, written informed consent is necessary. You must know and follow the laws in your state regarding HIV testing.

- Diagnostic uncertainty, particularly at later stages of HIV infection.
- Poor tolerability of antipsychotics at later stages of HIV infection.
- Overlap of metabolic side-effect profiles of ART and antipsychotics.
- Different treatment systems for medicinal and psychiatric illnesses.

A critically important factor in HIV care is optimal adherence to ART to prevent worsening of immune function and development of drug resistance. Major psychiatric factors that lead to poor adherence with ART in HIV-infected patients are depression and *active* substance use, particularly cocaine use and alcohol. It is usually unwise to initiate ART if adherence is very unlikely. Uncontrolled psychosis is another situation in which it might be better to postpone treatment with ART. However, if a patient has advanced AIDS (CD4 cell count <200/mm^3), treatment should be started as soon as possible.

 TIP

Initiation of ART is generally not a medical emergency. Optimal adherence is important to achieving successful outcomes, and time spent to identify and remove barriers to adherence at the beginning of treatment is time well spent.

When a patient with schizophrenia and known HIV infection worsens psychiatrically, it is important to consider medical causes of psychosis before assuming that the psychosis is part of the natural course of schizophrenia. The differential diagnosis of psychosis in an HIV-infected patient is rather lengthy, and in any patient with advanced AIDS, organic causes must be ruled out first (Table 22.1). By contrast, in a patient with well-controlled HIV disease (e.g., CD4 count >350/mm^3 and undetectable viral load), organic causes of psychosis are not as likely as the usual offenders (i.e., antipsychotic nonadherence, illicit drug or alcohol use, or the natural fluctuation of symptoms), but you still should keep in mind the possibility of an HIV-related illness as the cause for psychosis. Rarely, in patients with advanced AIDS, HIV encephalitis or dementia can present with psychotic symptoms and lead to diagnostic confusion if there is no history available.

TABLE 22.1. **Differential Diagnosis of Psychosis in HIV-Positive Patients with Schizophrenia**

HIV encephalitis
HIV dementia
HIV-related opportunistic infections
HIV medication-induced psychosis (unlikely on stable ART regimen)
Non-HIV–related intercurrent medical illness
Drug-induced psychosis
Exacerbation of schizophrenia due to nonadherence
Natural fluctuation of schizophrenia (even with treatment)

The treatment with antipsychotics is often uncomplicated, with two exceptions: drug interactions and motor side effects. As a rule of thumb, regimens based on non-nucleoside reverse transcriptase inhibitors (NNRTIs) and protease inhibitors (PIs) are potentially problematic with regard to pharmacokinetic drug interactions since they interact with CYP 3A4 (which metabolizes all antipsychotics to some degree). Of the NNRTIs, efavirenz and nevirapine induce 3A4, which can lead to antipsychotic failure—watch out for psychotic relapse. All PIs and the third NNRTI, delavirdine, inhibit 3A4, which can lead to increased antipsychotic serum levels—watch out for dose-related side effects. In my experience, patients with HIV disease who have schizophrenia tolerate and require the usual doses of antipsychotics; most patients that I treat receive second-generation antipsychotics. It is concerning that the side-effect profile of many antiretroviral medications and second-generation antipsychotics is similar: For example, glucose intolerance and dyslipidemia are common side effects of many of the drugs used to treat HIV and psychosis. In later disease stages, patients are more susceptible to extrapyramidal side effects. Another potential overlapping toxicity is bone marrow suppression due to the antiretroviral agent zidovudine (azidothymidine [AZT]) and agranulocytosis associated with clozapine. However, in HIV patients with schizophrenia whose psychosis is refractory to other antipsychotics (or who are very sensitive to extrapyramidal side effects), clozapine might be the only option and should be offered under close supervision.

Despite many theoretical and practical problems, treatment of HIV in patients with schizophrenia is often successful, particularly in those patients who by nature of the severity and chronicity of their mental illness are well

TABLE 22.2. SPMI and HIV—The Role of the Psychiatrist

Detect HIV infection—Screen and assess for risk factors

Prevent HIV infection or spread of infection—Education and skills training

Link patients to HIV treatment and advocate for optimal treatment of HIV

Coordinate care with medicine—Identify and treat psychiatric obstacles to successful ART

connected to psychiatric and medical services and live in supervised settings. Adding HIV treatment poses fewer difficulties than usually expected, and studies have shown similar rates of ART initiation and persistence between HIV patients with or without schizophrenia. This is important to know and should be conveyed to medical teams if there is hesitation to initiate treatment for a patient because of his or her psychiatric diagnosis. However, a group of so-called "triply diagnosed" patients—HIV infection, SPMI, and drug use—poses particular challenges in treatment engagement and adherence. Possible roles for psychiatrists in the treatment of HIV-infected patients with schizophrenia are outlined in Table 22.2.

ADDITIONAL RESOURCES

Web Sites

http://www.hopkins-aids.edu—The world-renowned Johns Hopkins AIDS Service.

http://www.thebodypro.com—The professional section of one of the most comprehensive HIV resources for patients, The Body.

http://www.psych.org/AIDS—The American Psychiatric Association AIDS Resource Center.

Book

Treisman GJ, Angelino AF. *The psychiatry of AIDS: A guide to diagnosis and treatment*. Baltimore: Johns Hopkins University Press; 2004.—A very accessible book on psychiatric care of HIV patients by one of the fathers of HIV psychiatry, Glenn Treisman.

Article

Branson BM, Handsfield HH, Lampe MA, et al. Revised recommendations for HIV testing of adults, adolescents, and pregnant women in health-care settings. *MMWR Recomm Rep.* 2006;55(RR14):1–17.—The new CDC recommendations regarding universal HIV testing.

23   **Dual Diagnosis**

Essential Concepts

- "Dual diagnosis" patients, as discussed in this chapter, are patients with schizophrenia who also suffer from a drug or alcohol use disorder. Half of patients with schizophrenia have a current or past problem with drugs or alcohol.
- Alcohol and cannabis use disorders are the most common comorbidities after nicotine.
- Given the scope of the problem, screen all patients with schizophrenia for substance use, including for "low-grade" use that is nevertheless impairing.
- Treatment is most successful if concurrent and integrated, that is, the patient receives treatment in one system.

"Bacchus hath drowned more men than Neptune."
—*Thomas Fuller, British physician and adage collector,*
1654–1734

"Dual diagnosis" denotes the co-occurrence of a psychiatric condition, in our case schizophrenia, and a drug or alcohol use disorder. The term is neither precise (other dual diagnoses exist, for example, mental illness with developmental disorders) nor does it delineate a homogeneous class of patients (different mental disorders ranging from anxiety disorders to psychosis combined with any use to dependence), but the term has stuck. It came into being when, in the 1980s, a new cohort of "young adult chronic patients" who had never been institutionalized overwhelmed a treatment system that was ill-prepared to treat poorly compliant, drug-misusing patients with schizophrenia in the community, leading to the phenomenon of revolving-door psychiatric admissions.

KEY POINT

Although the term "dual diagnosis" captures the problem of rather significant comorbidity, the term is not a diagnosis with specific interventions. Each of the disorders present in "dual" contributes to the outcome independently, and needs to be diagnosed and treated optimally and specifically in its own right.

In this chapter, I am discussing substance use in patients with diagnosed schizophrenia; the diagnostic difficulties that arise regarding drug-induced psychosis versus schizophrenia are dealt with in a separate chapter (Chapter 4). Smoking is so common and its consequences so devastating that I devote the whole next chapter to nicotine dependence. Caffeine, another common comorbidity, deserves a brief mention. In moderation, caffeine can be useful to counteract drug-induced sedation. However, excessive caffeine use can cause caffeine intoxication ("caffeinism"). Consider caffeinism in your restless patient with sleep problems.

SCOPE OF THE PROBLEM

Already in their first episode of schizophrenia, 30% of patients have a substance use disorder (the exact percentage will vary with region and definition of substance use) (Larsen et al., 2006). Substance-misusing first-episode patients are typically young men, and they often have better premorbid social, but poorer academic, adjustment compared to their nonabusing counterparts. In the Clinical Antipsychotic Trials of Intervention Effectiveness (CATIE) cohort, which is more representative of chronic patients, almost 4 in 10 patients had a current substance use problem (Swartz et al., 2006). Lifetime rates of any substance use problem are even higher.

TIP

Epidemiology counts, literally and figuratively: As a rule of thumb, remember that at least half of your patients with schizophrenia have a lifetime problem with substance use, and about one quarter will have an active substance use disorder.

In the United States, alcohol and cannabis use are the most common problems among patients with schizophrenia. Cocaine use, and, interestingly, hallucinogen use, occurs with some frequency as well, whereas, curiously, opiate misuse seems to be infrequent to almost nonexistent. Know your particular epidemiologic situation (e.g., is methamphetamine or phenylcyclohexylpiperidine [PCP] use common in your community?) and the drug use patterns in your patient population (e.g., college students misusing prescription stimulants or party drugs, including ketamine).

Those with alcohol problems seem to have a worse prognosis because alcohol is quite simply a rather toxic substance if used excessively. It is interesting that despite the adverse consequences of drug use, patients with schizophrenia and drug use problems (other than alcohol) tend to look better with regard to negative symptoms, even though positive symptoms are exacerbated. This suggests some drugs either remedy a deficit (the "self-medication hypothesis") or that drug use flags those patients who have a better prognosis because they are less biologically impaired; you have to be more "with it" to be able to obtain the drugs.

Several epidemiologic studies suggest that cannabis use is especially problematic: Frequent premorbid cannabis use (i.e., more than 50 uses) increases the risk for the development of schizophrenia by sixfold (Andreasson et al. 1987). This is seen as evidence that—in susceptible patients—cannabis use can trigger psychosis.

Drug use can have devastating effects on patients, families, and society. Other than the obvious social (e.g., homelessness; drug-related crimes), legal (i.e., arrests), financial (i.e., compounding poverty), and medical (e.g., human immunodeficiency virus [HIV] which can lead to patients being "triply diagnosed" with HIV, a drug problem, and a psychiatric disorder) problems from drug use, drugs can maintain or cause psychiatric symptoms, and drug use is an important factor in psychotic relapse. One consequence of drug use is poorer compliance with treatment of? all its sequelae. Violence is much more likely if there is drug use.

ASSESSMENT

Given the prevalence of substance use in schizophrenia, screening all patients to *detect* substance use problems is important. All too often, significant substance use is either not recognized at all or its severity not acknowledged. Make sure you get collateral information and do not rely on self-report alone. Laboratory screening to help diagnose unrecognized problems is essential. Saliva drug testing for point-of-service use in the office, and hair testing for drugs ingested in the previous 3 months are options to consider. Hair testing poses its own problems—depending on the hair style in fashion (you need a sufficient amount).

Diagnostically, you have two problems. First, it can be next to impossible to disentangle the contributions to psychopathology from the primary disorder and from substances. In many cases, however, the longitudinal history will eventually clarify the diagnoses. Second, patients with schizophrenia lead different lives, and the usual screening questions and diagnostic categories do not necessarily work well: If you never worked or if you never married, you cannot lose your job or your marriage over drinking.

 TIP

Classify as "use with impairment" to indicate problematic use that does not reach the level of severity required for a drug abuse or dependence diagnosis. Even low-grade use can be devastating for vulnerable brains in vulnerable populations.

Try to figure out where your patient fits in a four-stage dual-diagnosis treatment model put forth by the pioneers in dual diagnosis research, Drs. Robert Drake and Kim Mueser:

- Engagement—Patients have no working relationship with a clinician
- Persuasion—Patients are in contact with clinicians, discussing substance use
- Active treatment—Patients are working to reduce or cease substance use
- Relapse prevention—Patients have not had problems related to substances for several months

CLINICAL VIGNETTE

You have known Emilian for 10 years after he moved to Boston from the West Coast "because of the weather." In his 50s now, he is reliable in his clinic visits and takes an antipsychotic for schizophrenia. He lives in an apartment and does some volunteer work. One day, he does not show up for his monthly appointment. To your surprise, you learn that he was found drunk in an alley and admitted to a hospital, acutely psychotic. After his discharge, he tells you for the first time that he had a severe alcohol problem in his 30s but thought "I had it under control." He started drinking again a few months ago and had stopped his antipsychotic for fear of "an interaction."

The moral in this vignette is that epidemiology counts, literally and figuratively: The odds for a lifetime substance use history are 50:50. Unfortunately, relapse remains a lifelong [MW] possibility for any substance use disorder, and preventing alcohol relapse became an important focus of treatment in Emilian's case. Naltrexone and a referral to Alcoholics Anonymous (AA) helped re-establish sobriety.

TREATMENT

Probably the most important insight gained over the past decades has been that both the addiction and the psychiatric disorder need to be treated simultaneously, preferably in an integrated setting. This means that your patients are probably better off if you are comfortable providing all their psychopharmacology and if your own clinic also offers the psychosocial services necessary to address substance use (e.g., assertive outreach, case management, supported housing). Many psychosocial programs need to be modified to take into account the cognitive problems that often accompany schizophrenia. However, higher-functioning patients can successfully take advantage of? community support programs like 12-step programs (e.g., AA).

Meet your patients where they are: If abstinence is unrealistic, work on harm reduction. Contingency management (e.g., payeeship) can work well to motivate patients to learn skills to change substance use behaviors. Expect that treatment needs to be provided (and closely monitored) for many years for incremental learning to occur.

Pharmacologic treatment of the addiction is ancillary to the psychosocial treatments, never the only treatment. The antidipsomanic medication naltrexone (ReVia) at a dose of 50 mg per day can be safely used in alcoholic patients with schizophrenia. Naltrexone has become available as a once-a-month injectable form (Vivitrol), which eliminates the need to take (and remember) pills. I stay away from disulfiram (Antabuse) because of some reports of psychosis and its potential dangerousness if alcohol is consumed despite taking disulfiram. I am unsure which patient can reliably take the third available antidipsomanic, acamprosate (Campral), which has to be taken three times daily (two 333-mg pills tid). With regard to antipsychotics in dually diagnosed patients, consider the following points:

- Long-acting antipsychotics can help avoid treatment interruption during times of drug use.
- Clozapine seems to have unique efficacy to reduce substance use in schizophrenia.
- Cocaine increases a patient's risk for dystonia, neuroleptic malignant syndrome, and priapism; cocaine might be particularly dangerous with clozapine.

Last, as George Vaillant, a Harvard psychiatrist who studies adult development, including recovery from alcoholism, put it, getting a life (back) together requires more than not using a substance. See Chapter 20 on rehabilitation for more on this point.

ADDITIONAL RESOURCES

Book

Dennison SJ. *Handbook of the dually diagnosed patient: Psychiatric and substance use disorders.* Philadelphia: Lippincott Williams & Wilkins; 2003.—A very practical handbook of dual diagnosis that includes chapters on schizophrenia.

24 ▼ Nicotine Dependence

Essential Concepts
- Seven of ten patients with schizophrenia smoke. Many smokers with schizophrenia are severely addicted to nicotine.
- Assist smoking patients with schizophrenia in smoking cessation to reduce cardiovascular mortality and lung diseases. Make smoking cessation an explicit treatment goal.
- Most patients with schizophrenia will need maximum treatment with nicotine replacement therapy (NRT) and bupropion to successfully quit.
- Successful smoking cessation and relapse prevention require modified and probably long-term treatment compared to standard approaches.
- Smoking accelerates the metabolism of antipsychotics, particularly olanzapine and clozapine.

"It's easy to quit smoking. I've done it hundreds of times."
—*Mark Twain, 1835–1910*

The majority of patients with schizophrenia smoke, often prior to onset of psychosis. In a typical community mental health center, you can expect that 7 of 10 patients with schizophrenia smoke, a conservative estimate. Patients with schizophrenia are heavy smokers (often >20 cigarettes/day), suggesting that many patients are severely addicted to nicotine. Smoking is not only one of the Framingham risk factors for heart disease, but it also causes a host of smoking-related lung diseases that can lead to early death or reduce quality of life (e.g., chronic obstructive pulmonary disease).

Traditionally, smoking was seen to be part of the mental health culture; the smoke break continues to be part of many hospital routines to combat boredom. Mental health counselors who smoked saw smoking with patients as an opportunity for engagement rather than as a problem. Some remain confused about the potential benefits of smoking in this population, such as calming patients or treating a presumed nicotinic deficit. As a result, nicotine dependence has not been addressed as vigorously in this patient population as in the rest of society. This attitude is changing, albeit slowly.

 KEY POINT

See smoking as the threat it is for your patients, both in terms of health risk but also as a financial disaster if patients spend more than one third of their income on cigarettes. Psychiatrists, with their expertise in addictions and their frequent visits with patients compared to primary care, are ideally positioned to take the lead in smoking cessation.

I cannot overemphasize the pernicious effects of low expectations. From social science research, we know that nothing is more effective in creating poor outcomes than low expectations. I have been taught by many patients with schizophrenia that smoking cessation is possible, even in cases that seemed beyond hope. As Mark Twain recognized, sustained abstinence requires more than one attempt—on average, five attempts in ex-smokers from the general population. It is, however, incorrect to claim that severely addicted patients with schizophrenia do as well with smoking cessation as normal control-population cohorts. In some patients, harm reduction (smoking less) might be all that can be accomplished in a given quit attempt. Smoking less, however, can lead to compensatory smoking with higher exposure to carbon monoxide (CO) and carcinogens. The literature is also pointing toward higher relapse rates in patients with schizophrenia once pharmacologic smoking cessation treatment is withdrawn, indicating that some degree of treatment might have to be provided on an ongoing basis (Evins et al., 2005).

SMOKING CESSATION—BASICS

To help, you must first identify your smokers. At the initial visit, obtain a good smoking history (age of first smoking, amount of current smoking, previous quit attempts, longest duration of previous abstinence, smoking-related health problems). As part of every follow-up office visit, assess the patient's amount of smoking and willingness to quit. Although this might seem excessive, it is nevertheless useful for patients to know that, as their psychiatrist, you take smoking seriously and have made smoking cessation a treatment goal.

 TIP

Record smoking status (e.g., 1 pack per day) in every patient chart. You might want to consider smoking status as a "vital sign."

The "five A's" of the Public Health Service guidelines are a useful framework for help with smoking cessation:

- Ask (about smoking)—"Do you smoke?" "Do you want to quit?"
- Advise—(against smoking and recommend quitting).
- Assess (readiness to quit)—"Are you interested in quitting within the next month?"
- Assist (with smoking cessation)—Refer to smoking cessation program and start treatment.
- Arrange (for follow-up)—See or call patient 1 week after quitting.

Routine referrals to general smoking cessation programs can be difficult for patients with schizophrenia, so you might have to provide counseling and support by using motivational interviewing techniques. One important principle of motivational interviewing is that you never argue for change, but let the patient come to the conclusion that change is not only possible but desirable. For this to occur, the benefits of quitting must outweigh the benefits of continuing to smoke; have a patient list the positive things about smoking, not just the negative things, to clarify this for patients. For long-term smokers, quitting can seem impossible. Intermediate, achievable goals, like temporary abstinence or a reduced number of cigarettes per day (or even simply delaying every cigarette by 20 minutes), not complete smoking cessation, are necessary and acceptable steppingstones to eventual commitment to quitting for good.

 TIP

Use motivational interviewing techniques to assess readiness to quit, and guide patients toward considering and preparing to quit (e.g., have patient make list of benefits from smoking, benefits from quitting, barriers to quitting—feared weight gain could be a considerable obstacle). It helps if you assign your patient to one of Prochaska and DiClemente's stages of change (i.e., precontemplation, contemplation, preparation, action, and maintenance/relapse) so you can select the stage-appropriate intervention (see WELL CARD Smoking Cessation—Stages of Change in Appendix C).

One thing you can do is calculate a patient's 10-year risk for a major cardiac event using Framingham risk scoring (see Additional Resources in Chapter 21 on how to do this). This might increase motivation to eliminate one major risk factor, smoking.

The "five R's" provide a useful framework for discussion to enhance motivation to quit:

- *Relevance:* Discuss the impact of tobacco use on health and family, and the associated social stigma. Help the patient understand why quitting would be personally important.
- *Risks:* Discuss negative tobacco consequences. Have the patient identify negative health consequences or risks that are personally important.
- *Rewards:* Discuss benefits of tobacco cessation (health, financial, energy-level increase, recovery, role model).
- *Roadblocks:* Ask about barriers to quitting. "What is the one thing that keeps you from quitting?"
- *Repetition:* Address cessation at each visit. Always remember that this is a process and that your patient can learn from each experience of quitting.

All patients who are interested in quitting should receive drug therapy to eliminate nicotine withdrawal and block the reinforcing properties of nicotine. In the general population, each treatment alone roughly doubles quit rates compared to placebo. If you only had two questions to ask your smoker who is about to quit, you can assess the degree of biologic nicotine dependence by asking the following questions taken from the "Fagerstrom," a widely used questionnaire in smoking research:

- "How soon after you wake up do you smoke your first cigarette?" (within 30 minutes)
- "How many cigarettes do you smoke per day?" (at least 20)

The degree of biologic dependence (resulting in withdrawal) is severe if more than 20 cigarettes are smoked and smoking is one of the first things done after waking up (within

30 minutes). Note that this might not be valid if smoking is not
ad lib (e.g., group home). The more severely addicted, the
more treatment will be necessary. For patients with schizophrenia, maximum pharmacologic treatment is probably the
way to go and, unless contraindicated, combination pharmacotherapy (bupropion plus patch, which act synergistically)
and probably high-dose nicotine replacement therapy (NRT;
patch plus gum/inhaler/spray) should be used. A new medication Varenicline (Chantix) has recently been approved for
smoking cessation. The basic outline of an 8-week to 12-week
drug treatment plan for smoking cessation is simple, and you
should be able to routinely help a patient set up an individualized plan (consult WELL CARD Smoking Cessation—Drug
Therapies in Appendix C for more details) (Rigotti, 2002):

- Set quit date.
- Start bupropion 1 week prior to quit date.
- Start patch on quit date (usually 21 mg) for 4 weeks, then
  14 mg for 2 weeks, then 7 mg for 2 weeks, then discontinue.
- Throughout, add gum or lozenges or nasal spray, as
  needed, for craving.
- Decide with patient how long to continue bupropion and
  prn NRT.

In general-population smoking cessation programs, NRT is
usually tapered and discontinued over 4 to 8 weeks. For
patients with schizophrenia, long-term treatment might be
needed as the relapse rates are rather high once treatment is
discontinued. If you can, monitor for abstinence to help prevent relapse, or intervene early (e.g., monitor expired CO or
cotinine levels in plasma, urine, or saliva).

SMOKING CESSATION—CLINICAL PROBLEMS

Smoking influences the metabolism of several antipsychotics.
Most affected are antipsychotics with significant 1A2 metabolism, that is, clozapine and olanzapine. On average, patients
are able to decrease by half their antipsychotic plasma level
when they smoke, as certain ingredients in tobacco smoke,
specifically polycyclic aromatic hydrocarbons (but not nicotine itself), induce 1A2. Smoking cannabis has effects similar
to smoking cigarettes with regard to enzyme induction. NRT,
which is merely nicotine, has no effect on 1A2. First-generation
antipsychotic levels are also significantly reduced in smokers,
possibly because smoking effects UGT, which plays some role

in antipsychotic metabolism. To complicate things, caffeine (many smokers drink a lot of coffee) has the opposite effect on 1A2; it blocks it (Table 24.1).

Enzyme induction can be important if patients are titrated up on an antipsychotic in a (smoke-free) hospital where they might have been receiving the patch. The antipsychotic dose has to be adjusted upward after discharge once patients resume smoking at home. Conversely, if patients successfully quit smoking, the antipsychotic dose can be lowered.

Smokers who are admitted to a hospital for medical or psychiatric reasons and are not allowed to smoke can experience nicotine withdrawal. Clearly, this must be addressed. Most hospitalizations are short enough that the P450 system is not affected, as the P450 enzymes take several weeks to reach their noninduced state.

Anticipate concerns, for example, weight gain and anxiety, that patients who are considering quitting will have and try to alleviate those. On average, patients who quit will gain up to 10 lb (compare this risk with 10 years of smoking 1 pack per day). Patients are used to thinking that nicotine is calming, whereas in reality it is anxiogenic (just ask any nonsmoker who tries a cigarette), and smoking simply alleviates the anxiety that comes from nicotine withdrawal.

Nicotine withdrawal is limited to about 2 weeks, and it can easily be treated with NRT. The signs and symptoms of nicotine withdrawal can be confused with a psychotic relapse:

- Dysphoria and irritability; anxiety
- Insomnia
- Lower heart rate
- Restlessness
- Difficulties concentrating

TABLE 24.1. Nicotine Facts

Nicotine	Half-life 2 hours	Half-life 24 hours
Primary metabolite	Cotinine[a]	
Metabolism	Major **2A6**	
	Minor 2B6; glucuronidation	
Smoking induces 1A2 (and probably other enzyme systems, including UGT)		

[a]Cotinine is a useful marker of tobacco smoking. Cotinine can be measured in plasma, urine, or saliva.

ADDITIONAL RESOURCES

Web Sites

http://www.cdc.gov/tobacco—The smoking and tobacco use site put out by the Centers for Disease Control and Prevention. http://www.surgeongeneral.gov/tobacco—Look under the Clinician Section for "Treating Tobacco Use and Dependence—Clinical Practice Guideline" and "Treating Tobacco Use and Dependence—Clinician's Packet." From the Department of Health and Human Services.

Article

Mallin R. Smoking cessation: Integration of behavioral and drug therapies. *Am Fam Physician*. 2002;65:1107–1114.—Summary of smoking cessation for primary care physicians.

Refractory Psychosis and Clozapine

Essential Concepts

- Not all patients with schizophrenia have a meaningful response to antipsychotics: 1 patient in 4 benefits little from first-line antipsychotics; 1 in 10 has no response at all to any antipsychotic, including clozapine.
- Make sure you are not dealing with "pseudo-refractoriness": wrong diagnosis or missed diagnoses, unrecognized adherence problem, or drug use.
- Before switching, optimize the dose of the antipsychotic that the patient is already taking.
- Consider a (time-limited) clozapine trial after two failed, adequate antipsychotic trials; one of the antipsychotics should have been olanzapine.

> "The tragedy of life is what dies inside a man while he lives."
> —*Albert Schweitzer, 1875–1965, Nobel Prize for Peace 1952*

Most patients with schizophrenia have a meaningful reduction in positive symptoms from first-line antipsychotics. Unfortunately, the tragedy of life, to paraphrase Schweitzer, leaves 20% to 30% of patients treatment refractory, with little to no symptomatic response to first-line antipsychotics. Some estimate that 10% of patients with schizophrenia have no response whatsoever to any antipsychotic, including clozapine.

I will call "refractory" those patients who do not have a clinically meaningful reduction in impairing positive symptoms despite two adequate (in dose and duration) antipsychotic trials. In this definition, clozapine is not counted toward refractoriness. Note that while the definition I use refers to positive symptoms, functional impairment is implied. Patients who are refractory to clozapine fall into a category by themselves. It is, of course, the illness that is refractory, not the patient; put differently, it is our treatment that is ineffective for a patient.

CLINICAL APPROACH FOR REFRACTORY PSYCHOSIS

When faced with a poor medication response, ask yourself three questions:

1. Is the patient truly refractory, or are you dealing with "pseudo-refractoriness"?
2. Is your currently prescribed regimen adequate and optimized?
3. Has the patient had several, well-conducted sequential antipsychotic trials?

Rule out "Pseudo-refractoriness"

Before you label a patient refractory, make sure that you have ruled out the following three problems that can contribute to an apparent poor medication response:

1. Wrong and/or missed diagnoses
2. Drug misuse
3. Partial adherence or nonadherence

Comorbid drug use is probably one of the more common reasons for a poor response. If there is any chance that partial adherence might be the problem, consider a time-limited trial of a long-acting antipsychotic to clarify the issues. There is the additional possibility that some patients respond better to this type of "smooth" drug delivery compared to the intermittent spiking from oral dosing.

 TIP

Recommend a time-limited trial of a long-acting, injectable antipsychotic to eliminate the possibility of partial adherence if you cannot be sure about sufficient adherence.

A mistaken assumption of refractoriness has grievous consequences. It leads to polypharmacy, higher than necessary medication doses, poor treatment choices, and more side effects. Patients with intermittent compliance do not get used to side effects, and they might even run the risk of dangerous problems from starting a medication at full dose after missing a week of medications. Mistaken assumption of nonresponse to a particular medication can lead the clinician to giving up on a potentially valuable medication for the rest of that patient's life.

Optimize Current Regimen

Assuming you are confident that your diagnosis is correct and that neither drug misuse nor partial adherence is to blame for continuing symptoms, review your currently prescribed treatment: Is it adequate in duration and optimized in dose?

The duration of an adequate trial depends on the clinical situation and cannot be boiled down to one number. You should expect some clearly detectable clinical response after 4 to 6 weeks of treatment (not counting a titration period). If there is no response at all after 4 to 6 weeks, I would probably switch treatment earlier rather than later, particularly if symptoms are severe. If there is a clear response, it is important to allow symptoms to resolve and not switch prematurely: Time on medication is as important as the dose of medication since psychosis needs to be given time to resolve. Similarly, functional benefits of adequate symptom control will accrue only with time. Giving more medication cannot accelerate this process. It is a mistake to "push the dose" after 1 week of hospitalization, with little change in core psychotic symptoms. In other words, optimizing a medication can mean decreasing the dose or adding something to counteract side effects. Many patients will in fact often show some signs of improvement as early as week 1 (e.g., in sleep, in agitation). It is simply unrealistic to expect the resolution of delusions during a brief hospitalization.

Some patients might require a higher antipsychotic dose because of smoking, drug interactions (e.g., somebody on carbamazepine), or idiosyncrasies in drug metabolism.

 TIP

Consider checking antipsychotic serum levels in unclear situations. A nondetectable antipsychotic level at the usual dose suggests either an adherence problem or unusual metabolism.

For some but not all antipsychotics, a higher than usual dose can lead to further improvement (see Table 11.3). This is not true for first-generation antipsychotics and risperidone, for which pushing the dose buys you only more side effects. In some situations, reducing the dose might be more useful, for example, if akathisia is adding insult to injury. There is also no clear rational or clinical trial evidence why pushing aripiprazole beyond 15 to 20 mg per day should be an effective strategy. The only antipsychotic for which a higher-than-approved dose has been shown to be useful is olanzapine (shown for a dose of up to 30 mg/day; Volavka et al., 2002). Ziprasidone as currently approved (up to 160 mg/day;) might be underdosed, and some clinicians use up to 320 mg per day.

 TIP

Before giving up on olanzapine, consider an olanzapine trial at a dose of 30 mg per day. Note that this dose is higher than the Food and Drug Administration (FDA)-approved dose of 20 mg per day.

Conduct Sequential Antipsychotic Trials

The goal of sequential antipsychotic trials is not only to find an antipsychotic that might be more effective (and better tolerated) than another but to move toward clozapine, if indicated. Although we lump antipsychotics together as first-generation and second-generation antipsychotics, the second-generation antipsychotics in particular are all sufficiently different that patients should receive sequential trials of several of them. One-size-fits-all does not apply to second-generation antipsychotics. This is different from first-generation antipsychotics for which there is little benefit from switching among them.

How many trials should be conducted before recommending clozapine? Most guidelines recommend two well-conducted trials of an antipsychotic before moving to clozapine for refractory patients. This is a good rule-of-thumb, although, as noted in the previous paragraph,? ["sequential trials of several of them"] I do not necessarily adhere to it. If the two antipsychotics have not included olanzapine, I will often try olanzapine first as it seems to be more effective than other first-line antipsychotics (Lieberman et al., 2005). I also hesitate to count aripiprazole (because it is a partial agonist and our clinical experience is limited with this drug class) and quetiapine (because of its transient and weak dopamine-2 [D_2]-binding, which could render it less effective for some patients) toward failed drug trials. Last, I like to have one of the trials be risperidone or a first-generation antipsychotic (with "tight" D_2-binding) for the occasional patient who has a better response to those drugs with a good track record for efficacy (at least you know what you get). Obviously, you do not have to conduct these trials yourself if you have a clearly documented history of previous trials, although often you will find yourself in a position in which you simply not know what was previously done and to what effect.

CLOZAPINE FOR REFRACTORY PSYCHOSIS

Clozapine is the most effective antipsychotic that we have. In one seminal study by Kane et al. (1988), clozapine led to some improvement in 30% of patients who were prospectively treated with at least two antipsychotics (at the time, first-generation antipsychotics) and judged refractory. The superiority of clozapine has been confirmed in many trials, most recently in the Clinical Antipsychotic Trials of Intervention Effectiveness (CATIE) cohort, which included patients who had failed second-generation antipsychotics (McEvoy et al., 2006).

 KEY POINT

Clozapine should be part of your treatment algorithm for patients with schizophrenia. Given its clearly established superior efficacy in refractory patients, it is inexcusable to not at least strongly recommend a trial for patients with insufficient response to other antipsychotics.

Clozapine Trial

In practice, many patients never receive clozapine even though they have had more than enough failed antipsychotic trials. Many patients will be wary of what they have heard about clozapine, its host of potential side effects, and the need for regular blood work. First, convince yourself that clozapine is the next step, and then convince the patient.

 TIP

I always tell patients that I recommend a *time-limited trial* of clozapine: Trying it does not mean taking it "for the rest of your life." It gives the patient some control, and might avert a refusal of a clozapine trial (which requires the cooperation of the patient).

With clozapine, dosing should be based on serum levels as you cannot predict serum levels from the clozapine dose. One study found that a clozapine serum level range of 200 to 300 ng per mL was as effective as 350 to 450 ng per mL (VanderZwaag et al., 1996). I try to reach an initial range of 200 to 300 ng per mL but increase the dose to above 450 ng per mL if there is no response. (Note that the serum level is based on clozapine levels alone, not the combined clozapine plus norclozapine level, even though both numbers are reported by most laboratories.) In the case of clozapine, which requires a lengthy titration period or treatment duration of several months can be necessary to judge its efficacy. In patients who respond to clozapine, you will have to judge if the improvement that you see is worth the added side-effect burden that often accompanies clozapine use.

CLINICAL VIGNETTE

A young man, Alfred, came to my clinic after over 2 years of treatment for schizophrenia without much improvement. He had initially received risperidone but was switched to quetiapine after a few weeks when he did not get better. When I evaluated him, he experienced constant Schneiderian First-Rank Symptoms, preventing him from reading and concentrating on what people were saying to him; the distractions were so severe that he had been unable to work even part-time. There was no drug use, and (despite lack of efficacy) he had faithfully taken his prescribed antipsychotic. I switched him to olanzapine, which reduced his positive symptoms to the point that he could work again. We then negotiated a time-limited trial of clozapine to see if his positive symptoms would completely remit. Because clozapine led to complete symptom remission, he opted to continue with clozapine despite the need for blood monitoring.

This story is unfortunately all too common; patients are left with residual symptoms of psychosis even though the most effective antipsychotics, olanzapine and clozapine, have not been tried (for 2 years Alfred was left on an antipsychotic that was ineffective for him). Importantly, do not reserve clozapine only for the most severely ill patients. For this patient, clozapine brought additional benefit. It is my personal view that you should treat schizophrenia only if you are able to offer clozapine trials to patients.

Clozapine Nonresponse

If your patient does not respond to clozapine, you are leaving the realm of evidence-based medicine and entering the art of medicine. If there is truly no response to clozapine, switch patients back to the previously best-tolerated regimen, but augment if you think there was some benefit. Clozapine augmentation strategies include combining antipsychotics (one combination with some research support is clozapine plus risperidone; make sure, however, to read Chapter 17 on polypharmacy) or adding other medication classes, e.g., mood stabilizers, particularly valproate and lamotrigine (Chapter 15). Although rarely used in schizophrenia today, electroconvulsive therapy (ECT) remains a treatment option for florid, unresponsive psychosis. A desperate trial of an old drug, reserpine, can sometimes work, particularly in an excited psychosis.

Sometimes a fine line is drawn between "snowing the patient" and "treating the patient." Overly aggressive use of medications with limited efficacy has many risks for the patient. On the other hand, undertreating a violent, out-of-control patient brings suffering not only to society but ultimately to the patient.

ADDITIONAL RESOURCES

Articles

Kane J, Honigfeld G, Singer J, et al. Clozapine for the treatment-resistant schizophrenic: A double-blind comparison with chlorpromazine. *Arch Gen Psychiatry.* 1988;45:789–796.—Read this one, as it is one of only a handful of truly seminal articles on schizophrenia.
Iqbal MM, Rahman A, Husain Z, et al. Clozapine: A clinical review of adverse effects and management. *Ann Clin Psychiatry.* 2003;15:33–48.—A clinical review of clozapine.

Negative Symptoms

Essential Concepts

- Negative symptoms are a core feature of schizophrenia; they have diagnostic and prognostic significance.
- Negative symptoms comprise two main clusters: reduced affective experiences/expression and amotivation.
- Avoid and treat secondary negative symptoms, particularly depression.
- Educate family members about negative symptoms to reduce undue pressure on the patient.

"Dementia Praecox consists of a series of clinical states which have as their common characteristic a peculiar destruction of the internal connections of the psychic personality with the most marked damage of the emotional life and volition."
—*Emil Kraepelin, from the 8th edition of his textbook (1913)*

In this chapter, we look at a nonpsychotic symptom cluster: negative symptoms. Negative symptoms are characterized by a loss or diminution of function: something is missing that you expect to be there. Missing is the independent drive, the curiosity about the world, and the boundless energy that we expect from young people. Missing are also the facial expressions and body language that we take for granted when we engage somebody in dialogue. Patients themselves can perceive the lackluster quality of their inner experiences. Both Emil Kraepelin (see epigraph) and Eugen Bleuler (recall that two of his four As of schizophrenia are autism and affectivity) recognized the centrality of these symptoms to the experience of schizophrenia. In 1980, Timothy Crow made a very influential distinction between type I (mainly positive symptoms) and type II (mainly negative symptoms, with poor response to antipsychotics) and schizophrenia. A modern conceptualization of negative symptoms includes five broad symptom domains, listed in Table 26.1.

As a less modifiable aspect of the schizophrenia syndrome, negative symptoms are more the essence of schizophrenia

TABLE 26.1. Negative Symptom Domains[a]

Alogia	Lack of words (poverty of speech or poverty of content of speech)
Blunted affect	Lack of affectivity (perception, experience, expression of emotions)
Anhedonia	Lack of capacity for pleasure
Avolition	Lack of volition ("will") and motivation
Asociality	Lack of social drive

[a]Terms based on National Institute of Mental Health–supported consensus conference (Kirkpatrick et al., 2006).

than positive symptoms, which can be seen as accessory (albeit key in defining psychotic disorders). It is rather obvious to any clinician that negative symptoms, unless mild, are profoundly impairing. "Will" is what keeps us going, and there is simply no substitute for it if it is missing.

The centrality of negative symptoms is now acknowledged and officially recognized in the DSM-IV as a core feature of schizophrenia, and two clinical subtypes of schizophrenia in which negative symptoms are the predominant feature have been described (Table 26.2). Negative symptoms can be a major factor in poor community functioning: imagine a person devoid of drive or capacity to experience reward and the clinical problems this poses with regard to rehabilitation, interpersonal functioning, or work. Clinically, the negative symptom domain,

TABLE 26.2. Schizophrenia Subtypes with Negative Symptoms

Deficit schizophrenia	Patients with prominent negative symptoms that are enduring and primary. Might be a subtype of schizophrenia with different risk factors (suggesting different etiology; Kirkpatrick et al., 2001). Depending on the chronicity of the patient sample, up to 30% will have the deficit syndrome.
Simple schizophrenia (officially recognized in ICD-10; called "simple deteriorative disorder" in DSM-IV research section)	Patients who never experienc positive symptoms but drift slowly into a withdrawn, empty mental state of essentially only negative symptoms.

rather than the cognitive domain, often seems to be the critical factor that determines community outcomes.

CLINICAL ASSESSMENT

Negative symptoms might not be obvious to the observer, but patients who can express their inner experiences will note that they have changed: things are harder; more mental effort is necessary to achieve the same results; previously enjoyable things are no longer exciting; they do not feel close to other people. In more severe cases, negative symptoms can be observed, and patients will appear blunted, disengaged from the world, and unable to participate in life beyond a very narrow area of immediate concern. Little is said either literally because patients are monosyllabic or because not much information is conveyed. Goal-setting is reduced (including, e.g., the simple goal of getting up and shaving). Patients fail projects because they do not persist.

 KEY POINT

Factor analysis suggests that the negative symptoms can be combined into two clusters: blunted affect and alogia form an emotional expressivity cluster; avolition, anhedonia, and asociality form an amotivation cluster (Kimhy et al., 2006).

These are some useful questions for assessing negative symptoms:

"Have you noticed a change in your emotions?" (*blunted affect*)
"What are your plans for this week?" (*avolition*)
"What gets you excited?" (*anhedonia*)
"When is the last time you did something with a friend?" (*avolition*)

Once you have identified the presence of negative symptoms, you are not quite done: Negative symptoms (just like a headache) are not a diagnosis. You now need to figure out why it is that you see negative symptoms (Table 26.3).

 TIP

An important distinction can sometimes be drawn between depression and negative symptoms. Although family members frame any withdrawal as "depression," some patients can distinguish between depression as a state of "suffering" and negative symptoms as a state of "emptiness." This distinction is not always clear, however.

TABLE 26.3. Differential Diagnosis of Negative Symptoms

Primary negative symptoms ("true" negative symptoms)
Secondary negative symptoms
  Depression and demoralization
  Positive symptoms
  Parkinsonism (bradyphrenia and bradykinesia)
  Sedation
  Lack of opportunity and stimulation (institutionalism)
  Social anxiety
  Severe cognitive problems (e.g., dementia, mental retardation)
  Neurologic apathy syndromes

Last, I want to note that although psychiatry owns the term "negative symptoms," negative symptoms are not specific to schizophrenia. Other specialties might simply have different words for it (e.g., the apathy syndrome seen in patients with Alzheimer disease or the abulia of neurology). Rating scales for negative symptoms can be applied to other patient groups, for example, patients with epilepsy or Alzheimer disease.

TREATMENT

The honest assessment is that we have no great specific treatments for primary negative symptoms. Social skills training is one psychosocial treatment that can help some patients. Pharmacologic treatments often have disappointingly little clinical impact on primary negative symptoms. Nevertheless, glycine agonists (e.g., D-cycloserine) are promising (but currently experimental), and other medication classes have some limited support (e.g., antidepressants or folate). While I remain unconvinced that antipsychotics can fundamentally treat primary negative symptoms, treatment with antipsychotics (in particular, second-generation antipsychotics) can improve negative symptoms, typically in parallel with an improvement in overall psychopathology (Buckley and Stahl, 2007). I acknowledge that I might be mistaken by dismissing such a response as merely treating secondary negative symptoms. You could even question the usefulness (and validity) of separating primary from secondary negative symptoms—how do I know what is primary and what is secondary? Certainly from the patient's perspective, it does not matter if a symptom is "primary" or "secondary." The distinction can nevertheless help organize your approach toward differential diagnosis, and I use it for this purpose.

Aggressively Treat Secondary Causes of Negative Symptoms

First, review all medicines and avoid those that cause or make negative symptoms worse. Offenders are all sedating medications and antipsychotics that cause parkinsonism (bradyphrenia or bradykinesia). It is rather difficult to get motivated if you are fighting daytime sleepiness. If you suspect parkinsonism, consider a switch to another antipsychotic (rather than adding an anticholinergic, which impairs cognition). Next, make sure that positive symptoms are optimally treated. Sometimes, unrecognized positive symptoms (e.g., paranoia) can lead you to falsely conclude that primary negative symptoms are present. Importantly, aggressively identify treatable psychiatric comorbidities such as social anxiety or depression.

CLINICAL VIGNETTE

I saw a young man in consultation 2 years after his first episode of psychosis had forced him to put his college education on hold. Although his psychosis had resolved with aripiprazole, he appeared rather blunted and he had been unable to return to college. He eloquently described a sense of loss of volition and a lack of emotional vividness. His Beck Depression Inventory II (BDI-II) depression score was only slightly elevated (total score of 15), but he considered himself somewhat depressed and unable to get motivated. I recommended a trial of an antidepressant for his residual affective and/or negative symptoms. When he returned for a follow-up visit 6 months later, I noted no change in his blunted appearance. However, his BDI-II total score was 2 and he considered himself recovered; he had taken up some classes at a local college.

Always consider the possibility of secondary negative symptoms, in this case, impairing subsyndromal depression. A self-rating scale for depression (e.g., the BDI) is useful (necessary) to identify and track subsyndromal symptoms. Another way of conceptualizing the clinical problem in the young man is to say that his anhedonia (a shared, core feature of both depression and negative symptoms) was antidepressant responsive, thus avoiding any academic discussions about what I was "really" treating.

Pace Yourself and the Family in Treating Negative Symptoms

Lack of environmental stimulation leads to a withering of social interest and competence (think about the deleterious effects of psychosocial neglect in orphanages). Without doubt, institutionalization adds to negative symptoms (note that patients can be neglected or "institutionalized in the community" as well). However, some families and patients push too hard and too early for patients to "get better." For some, negative symptoms appear to have a protective function (e.g., from overstimulation), and improvement follows its own trajectory and time course unless it is interfered with. There is a fine line between pushing too hard and doing too little.

 TIP

Spend time explaining negative symptoms and their impact on functioning to family members. Otherwise, patients are labeled as "lazy" and unrealistically pushed. Protect the patient from overly aggressive expectations; instead, stress the importance of giving time to heal. But do not have expectations that are unduly low.

ADDITIONAL RESOURCES

Article

Stahl SM, Buckley PF. Negative symptoms of schizophrenia: A problem that will not go away. *Acta Psychiatr Scand.* 2007;115:4–11. —A recent review on negative symptoms.

Cognition in Schizophrenia

27

Essential Concepts

- Cognitive deficits are a core feature of schizophrenia. How well a patient with schizophrenia will do in life is not determined by positive symptoms but in part by the degree of cognitive impairment.
- 75% of patients with schizophrenia are globally impaired across a broad range of neuropsychologic tests. Several areas are more affected than others, specifically attention, verbal memory, and executive function.
- The clock-drawing test is a good screening test for executive dysfunction, an area of poor function in more severely ill patients.
- Minimize medications that can hamper cognitions (in particular, anticholinergic medications and benzodiazepines).
- Minimize interventions that rely on verbal memory, an area of cognitive deficit in schizophrenia. Patients should rely on lists and routines.

> "Tell me and I'll forget; show me and I may remember; involve me and I'll understand."
> —*Author unknown*

Cognitive deficits are a core feature of schizophrenia. Kraepelin's term for schizophrenia, "dementia praecox," speaks to the early recognition that intellect and functional decline are important aspects of this disorder. Kraepelin also described patients with mental retardation who developed schizophrenia and for whom he used the term *Pfropfschizophrenie* (from the German *pfropfen*, "to graft on") to denote that the psychosis seems to have been grafted upon a malfunctioning brain. Kraepelin's thinking is reminiscent of today's neurodevelopmental model of schizophrenia that sees certain cognitive deficits as part of the vulnerability for schizophrenia.

The effects of cognitive impairments are devastating when it comes to function. Cognition predicts the ability to work, to participate in rehabilitation, or to function in the community. Real-life performance is complex, however, and while cognitive competence matters, significant negative symptoms (see previous chapter) are a second impediment to good community outcomes.

COGNITIVE IMPAIRMENTS IN SCHIZOPHRENIA

Cognitive impairments in schizophrenia are present before the onset of psychosis, possibly starting during puberty. Although there might be some worsening around the time of the first episode, the deficits plateau after the initial episode and probably remain stable throughout life. In other words, the cognitive damage is done once patients present with psychosis.

 KEY POINT

Although it is possible to be cognitively intact if you have schizophrenia, about 75% of patients would nevertheless be classified as impaired on standard, comprehensive neuropsychologic batteries (Palmer et al., 1997), sometimes reaching the level of dementia if the deficits encompass several cognitive domains and are severe enough.

Even those patients who are unimpaired on testing around the time of their first episode of psychosis probably have an illness-related decrement in their cognitive function. In one study, patients performed on average about 15 points lower on the IQ scale than expected.

On neuropsychologic testing, the pattern of impairment is described as both generalized (performance is impaired on a wide variety of tests) and specific (there is a typical pattern of impairment, with some areas more impaired than others) (Bilder et al., 2000). The biggest impairments are seen in the areas of attention (such as sustained attention or vigilance), verbal learning and memory, and executive function. In these key areas of cognition, patients show impairments between 1 and 1½ and 2 standard deviations below healthy controls. Social cognition, reasoning and problem solving, and speed of information processing are other cognitive domains that are usually measurably impaired.

A simplified neuroanatomical model of cognition in schizophrenia suggests that almost all patients have some problems with basic memory and learning (temporal–hippocampal system), coupled with executive dysfunction (prefrontal systems). The prefrontal dysfunction, in particular, prevents the use of organizational strategies to learn new material, which is necessary for effective learning. In Alzheimer disease, the memory problem is rather basic (the memory stores themselves are degraded); in schizophrenia, some aspects of the memory problem are at a higher level (where strategies and flexibility are needed for better access of memory stores). The cognitive problems of schizophrenia are unlike those of Alzheimer dementia or of typical "brain damage" in that the disease is neither progressive nor can the dysfunction be easily localized to one particular brain area, respectively. It is therefore better to think of impaired function (e.g., executive dysfunction) as opposed to impaired regions (e.g., frontal lobe dysfunction).

 KEY POINT

Although schizophrenia is clearly not a simple frontal lobe dementia, many patients have executive problems, and a minority have deficits akin to frontotemporal dementia with regard to severity and neuropsychologic profile (albeit not neuroanatomically) (de Vries et al., 2001).

CLINICAL ASSESSMENT

It should have become clear that any examination of a patient with schizophrenia is incomplete if you assess only positive and negative symptoms: You must also assess cognition. I stress this because cognition (despite being a core feature of the illness) is not included in current diagnostic criteria and might be overlooked, particularly because the deficits can be rather subtle and overshadowed by more obvious positive or negative symptoms. You should also know that the relationship between symptoms and cognition is not strong. Although there is some connection between negative symptoms and cognition (those with significant negative symptoms tend to have worse cognition), the correlation is rather weak ($r = 0.13$ to 0.27 in the Clinical Antipsychotic Trials of Intervention Effectiveness [CATIE] baseline data). Positive symptoms have essentially no correlation with cognition. In other words, you cannot really judge the severity of cognitive problems from the severity of symptoms.

Unfortunately, a good assessment of cognition is not easy as some areas of cognition require a computer or other equipment (and many tests are copyrighted). For some key domains (e.g., social cognition), no easy-to-use bedside test is clinically available. I suggest that you get your hands on some of the tests to look at the principle behind them and then create your own poor-man's version of them. For example, look at the Hopkins Verbal Learning Test (HVLT) and then create your own word list—you will need 12 words from three taxonomic categories; give a patient three trials to learn the list and see how the patient organizes learning.

 TIP

The most useful information might not come from the test results themselves but how a patient approaches a test, so it does not matter so much what exact test you use. What matters is that you administer the screening tests yourself to get an appreciation of the patient's cognitive struggles.

For a bedside assessment of cognition in schizophrenia, I suggest you examine the following key areas of cognition:

- Assess sustained attention/vigilance—Hard to test without a computer but a fundamental problem in schizophrenia; I use the digit span forward to make sure basic attention is okay.
- Assess working memory—Digit span backward and Trails B.
- Assess verbal learning and memory—Have patient learn a word list (e.g., based on HVLT, as mentioned above); look for poor memorization strategies that ignore semantic relationships, not absolute performance.
- Assess frontal lobe functions—This is a very important area to examine. At a minimum, have patient draw a clock. Table 27.1 presents other screening tests that you could use.
- Estimate processing speed—Trails A.
- Complete the Mini Mental State Examination (MMSE)—Note that the MMSE is not sufficient to assess cognition in patients with schizophrenia per se. A normal MMSE is useful information, as are the items on the MMSE that pose problems for the patient.

During the course of the interview, you should be able to form an opinion about the patient's IQ and ability to think in

TABLE 27.1. Bedside Assessment of Executive Function

Clock drawing[a]
Luria's hand maneuvers
Cognitive estimates
Verbal fluency—category fluency (supermarket items) and letter fluency (FAS)
Trails B

[a]If you only could do one test to check executive function do this one.

abstract terms. One of the best estimates of intelligence is a person's vocabulary (estimates of premorbid IQ use simple lists of words that have to be read aloud by patients and are scored based on correct pronunciation, for example, "terpsichorean"). Asking about similarities and the meaning of a proverb are good screening questions to determine ability to abstract. I prefer to ask proverbs that the patient does not know to see how the patient approaches the interpretation. Another way of gauging intelligence and practical thinking is the use of cognitive estimates: How high does an airplane fly? How tall is the Prudential (a tower in Boston—you obviously might want to choose a more local example)?

Remember that concrete thinkers do not benefit from abstract explanations. Do not be surprised if a concrete thinker resists a medication switch because the other medication requires a higher dose (e.g., 100 mg of quetiapine instead of 1 mg of risperidone).

Do not forget to ask about difficulties with reading, writing, spelling, and mathematics. A significant minority of patients are functionally illiterate but would never call themselves illiterate. A history of school problems could lead to a diagnosis of a specific learning disability that can accompany neurodevelopmental disorders. If a learning disorder is present, consider testing for velo-cardio-facial syndrome (VCFS).

 TIP

Routinely order comprehensive neuropsychologic testing (with emphasis on attention, memory, and executive functions) of your patient with schizophrenia to document areas of strength and weakness. I suggest doing testing once a patient is clinically stable and has reached a plateau, not during an acute illness phase. If you only could do one test, do the digit symbol coding task.

TREATMENT

Currently, no medications are available that can treat the cognitive impairment of schizophrenia. There was hope that the second-generation antipsychotics would have cognitive benefits over the first-generation antipsychotics. Unfortunately, it now seems more likely that antipsychotics have merely more or less liability toward further impairing cognition, in part related to dose and overall receptor profile. In one well-done study of antipsychotic-naïve, first-episode patients, risperidone was clinically effective but worsened already impaired spatial memory, likely an unintended (and unavoidable) consequence of the effect of antipsychotics on frontal dopamine systems (Reilly et al., 2006).

Do Not Add Insult to Injury

It is imperative to avoid further compromising an already compromised brain with alcohol, drugs, and medications, such as anticholinergics. Anticholinergic drugs, in particular, can worsen complex attention and memory in schizophrenia by 1 standard deviation (Minzenberg et al., 2004). I think it is rarely, if ever, justified to use a maintenance antipsychotic that requires the long-term addition of an anticholinergic. In those cases in which you have to start an anticholinergic, review the ongoing need for it a month after you start it (and try to lower the dose). Discourage diphenhydramine (Benadryl) for insomnia. Review your use of benzodiazepines, which also worsen memory function (but keep in mind the Yerkes–Dodson law and its inverted-U curve that posits an optimal amount of anxiety for performance, beyond which performance worsens).

Rely on Routines, Not on Memory

Recall one fundamental problem that many patients with schizophrenia have: verbal memory. If patients have problems with verbal memory, talking is not the best approach, and verbal repetition is not the best strategy for memory consolidation. Patients should not rely on their memory but write things down and use lists. However, the best way of learning for patients with schizophrenia is by doing through creating routines (using implicit memory) as understood by the writer of the proverb at the beginning of this chapter. Also note that many patients with schizophrenia have reading impairment that leaves them functionally illiterate.

Acknowledge Executive Dysfunction

If there is executive dysfunction, patients need somebody to substitute for them in those areas in which they have difficulties: planning ahead and implementing plans. Executive dysfunction becomes obvious when patients are left to their own devices (e.g., patients who had lived with their parents might be unable to function alone in college).

ADDITIONAL RESOURCES

Web Site

http://www.matrics.ucla.edu—Official MATRICS web site. MATRICS stands for Measurement and Treatment Research to Improve Cognition in Schizophrenia, an initiative by the National Institute of Mental Health (NIMH) to stimulate the development of drugs to improve cognition in schizophrenia.

Book

Harvey PD, Sharma T. *Understanding and treating cognition in schizophrenia: A clinician's handbook*. London: Martin Dunitz; 2002.—Concise and readable volume for clinicians.

28 ▼ Depression and Suicide

Essential Concepts
- Schizophrenia is a disease with at least 5% mortality: you can die *from* it young, not merely *with* it in old age. The cause of death is suicide.
- Most suicides by patients with schizophrenia occur in the first few years after diagnosis.
- Risk factors for suicide in schizophrenia are the known risk factors for suicide in other conditions: particularly drug use, depression or demoralization; and psychosis itself.
- Depression is common in schizophrenia, particularly in the early years of the illness.
- Demoralization can occur early in the course of illness as well if the illness does not get better and its ramifications on a patient's life become obvious to the patient.
- Clozapine reduces suicidality in schizophrenia.
- Schizophrenia brings many elements of caring for patients with chronic illness into sharp focus, particularly when patients become demoralized when their symptoms do not improve. The treatment of demoralization is giving hope. This requires your time and commitment.

> "There is but one truly serious philosophical problem, and that is suicide. Judging whether life is or is not worth living amounts to answering the fundamental question of philosophy."
> —*Albert Camus ("The Myth of Sisyphus"), 1942*

> "The most serious of schizophrenic symptoms is the suicidal drive."
> —*Eugen Bleuler, 1911*

The early prognosis in schizophrenia *quo ad vitam* ("with regard to life") is largely determined by suicide. Suicide is, in fact, the number one cause of premature death in schizophrenia.

The great Swiss psychiatrist Eugen Bleuler recognized suicide as a key clinical concern at a time when psychiatrists were just beginning to study schizophrenia. Today, we can only imagine how much some patients must have suffered in Bleuler's time when incessant, unrelenting auditory hallucinations drove them to suicide to silence the voices, as no treatment was available to quell them.

Most modern studies suggest that around 5% of patients diagnosed with schizophrenia die from suicide (Palmer et al., 2005). Although most practitioners recognize that schizophrenia is disabling, it is often not considered to be potentially lethal, so we need to focus on this important statistic: Schizophrenia is a disease with 5% mortality. You can die *from* schizophrenia as opposed to merely dying *with* it in old age. This risk of death from suicide is comparable to that of patients with primarily depressive disorders and many potentially lethal medical disorders.

Suicide attempts are even more prevalent than completed suicides. As many as half of the patients with schizophrenia that you encounter will have attempted suicide. This suicide risk is not stable over a patient's life. The risk is greatest in the first few years of the illness. Accordingly, most suicides occur in the first several years following diagnosis. However, suicide can occur at any time point. In longstanding schizophrenia, another risk factor for suicide is hospitalization. The risk of suicide increases shortly before going to the hospital (while acutely ill), while the patient is in the hospital, and shortly after discharge, particularly if the patient is socially isolated.

RISK FACTORS FOR SUICIDE

What mediates suicidality in schizophrenia? Importantly, most risk factors are the same as the risk factors in other patient populations, namely substance use, depression, and psychosis.

The first risk factor you should evaluate is substance use because of its effect on impulse control and mood.

The next risk factor you should consider is depression, which occurs often in the course of schizophrenia (Hafner et al., 2005). Depressive symptoms are very common in early-course schizophrenia. Further, a period of depression can coincide with or follow the resolution of positive symptoms, when patients are getting better. Such depressive symptoms and syndromes in the setting of improving or residual schizophrenia are sometimes called "post-psychotic depression," an admittedly poorly defined entity without clear time boundaries, severity definitions, or neurobiologic understanding. In addition to this purported connection to resolving or resolved psychosis, patients can develop a depressive episode at any point in their lives. Schizophrenia does not render one immune from depression.

The third key risk factor you should focus on is psychosis itself. Although probably less common today compared to the days of Bleuler, uncontrolled psychotic symptoms can still be responsible for unbearable psychologic pain (or psychache, as the father of American suicidology, Edwin Shneidman, calls it), leading to suicide attempts. Though you might think that so-called command hallucinations should be responsible for suicides, clinical studies suggest that this is true for a small minority of patients (about 10%), but not for most. Some psychotic patients die by accident in response to hallucinations or delusions. I treated a patient who jumped off a bridge not because he wanted to die, but in response to God's voice asking him, as a test of faith, to jump to prove his worthiness.

 TIP

Make sure you understand a patient's acute mental suffering: his or her "psychache." This psychache might come from acute psychosis or from clinical depression with its distorted self-loathing and gloomy views; from hopelessness. The psychache can be made worse by anxiety, which could stem from your treatment, in the form of akathisia. Relieve acute suffering acutely by treating aggressively with medications.

The patient's emotional and cognitive response to receiving a diagnosis of schizophrenia is also important. Receiving a (stigmatizing) diagnosis of schizophrenia is traumatic. The diagnosis brings fear and leads to a severe feeling of loss: the loss of one's future and standing in society. The way people see themselves and their role in society matters greatly. Imagined or real social exclusion can lead to a state of alienation and lack of purpose in life, which can result in what sociologists call *anomic suicide*. This seems to be particularly relevant for those patients who develop a good understanding of their predicament and its consequences, particularly if they had good academic achievements before the onset of schizophrenia. They are often the most intact patients who, in theory, have the best chances of substantial recovery and good long-term outcome.

Having "insight-into-illness" turns out to be a double-edged sword: insight is generally helpful in active disease management, but it might increase the suicide risk (Crumlish et al., 2005). Conversely, patients who are unaware of their symptoms, who are not bothered by their disability, and who have little understanding of their predicament are probably at lower risk for suicide.

⟁ KEY POINT

Demoralization is the loss of hope and loss of meaning and purpose in life. Demoralized people feel isolated from people and society. Demoralization is not the same as depression, although they can come together and there is some obvious overlap. One of the hallmarks of demoralization is a complaint of suicidality. The treatment for demoralization is giving hope and decreasing isolation.

Good questions for you to ask to tap into demoralization are as follows:

What do you want to accomplish over the next year?
What are your hopes for the future?
You have your whole life in front of you; what do you want to do with the time?

ASSESSMENT OF SUICIDALITY

It is important that you routinely assess suicidal ideation and monitor depression and demoralization when you treat patients with schizophrenia. Your assessment of suicidality should follow general clinical guidelines; the process is not different for schizophrenia except that you take into account schizophrenia-specific risks (e.g., demographics). I use "The ABCs of suicide" to comprehensively review important clinical data that go into my suicide risk assessment (see EM CARD Suicide Assessment in Appendix A for this checklist).

In addition to a good clinical assessment, the severity of suicidality and depression should be assessed with a rating scale, so both can be followed longitudinally and so that the response to treatment can be judged.

TIP

Keep track of depressive symptoms and suicidality with a rating scale. A well-validated rating scale for depression in schizophrenia is the Calgary Depression Scale for Schizophrenia (CDSS; see under Additional Resources). This scale is constructed in a way that avoids mistakenly rating negative symptoms as evidence for depression. Items that overlap in both conditions (e.g., anhedonia) are not included. Alternatively, a self-rating scale, such as the widely used Beck Depression Inventory (which contains an item on suicidality), can easily be integrated into routine clinical care. Although I strongly advocate using rating scales, no rating scale score can substitute for clinical judgment.

TREATMENT OF SUICIDALITY

Psychopharmacologic treatment with the goal of symptom control is often helpful, although this can, of course, only be true for those patients who accept your treatment. Suicides seem to occur more frequently in those with schizophrenia who remain untreated or who are insufficiently treated. This makes nonadherence and partial adherence risk factors for suicide.

In patients who present for treatment, maximum treatment of positive symptoms and active psychosis is the mandatory first step. While doing this, avoiding side effects that compound a patient's psychache, particularly akathisia, is important. Consider a clozapine trial if patients remain symptomatic: Clozapine is not only the most effective antipsychotic for positive symptoms, but also has the lowest liability for drug-induced dysphoric states like akathisia. In addition, it turns out that clozapine reduces suicidality. An international landmark trial, InterSePT (which stands for "International Suicide Prevention Trial") showed (using a randomized design) that clozapine can reduce suicidal behavior and suicide attempts in schizophrenia by about one quarter when compared with olanzapine (Meltzer et al., 2003).

Because of the strength of this finding, clozapine was subsequently approved by the Food and Drug Administration for recurrent suicidal behavior in schizophrenia, the only drug that carries this indication. The suicide-protective mechanisms might be severalfold, not mutually exclusive, including better symptom control, fewer extrapyramidal side effects, and less impulsivity. I would add, though, that about half the patients in the trial received antidepressants in addition to their assigned antipsychotic. Clozapine alone might therefore not be sufficient to treat depression and suicidality in schizophrenia. Some have pointed out that the choice of olanzapine as the comparator drug might have watered down clozapine's true efficacy, as olanzapine has some properties similar to clozapine. In fact, there was no difference in *completed* suicides between the olanzapine and clozapine arm in the InterSePT trial.

One problem with administering clozapine for suicidality is that those patients at the highest risk for suicide are early in the course of their illness and rarely receive clozapine because other antipsychotics are tried first. By the time clozapine is considered, it might be too late. I wonder sometimes if I should be more aggressive and move to clozapine earlier, rather than later, despite the risks of clozapine treatment. This is one of the truly difficult clinical decisions, and I usually end up trying olanzapine before moving on to clozapine.

🔖 TIP

Consider a trial of clozapine earlier, rather than later, for suicidal patients with schizophrenia. Clozapine might have a direct effect on the neurobiology of the "suicidal drive." It also works better for positive symptoms and causes less distressing neuroleptic-induced dysphoria.

One last thought on reducing suicidality with psychotropics: giving lithium to a patient with bipolar disorder can be life-saving. Unfortunately, lithium is not effective for the core symptoms of schizophrenia. Nevertheless, in more episodic forms of psychosis with significant mood components, it is reasonable to try lithium as an add-on therapy.

If depressive symptoms are present in the florid, acute phase of psychosis, antidepressants are probably not necessary. Depressive symptoms will recede as psychosis recedes. An older piece of literature even suggests that antidepressants given during this phase might hinder a therapeutic response. Although it is a common clinical problem, the pharmacologic management of depressive symptoms in the postacute phase of psychosis is surprisingly poorly studied. There seems to be a rather high placebo-response rate to antidepressants in this phase. Nevertheless, I would clearly treat syndromal presentations of major depression and chronic forms of depression (e.g., dysthymic disorder) with an added antidepressant, once the acute phase is over and positive symptoms are well controlled. This assumes that I have ruled out nonadherence to the antipsychotic medication, drug use, and extrapyramidal side effects that can look like depression.

⚜ KEY POINT

Although a cure is not always possible, treatment that alleviates suffering is. Accepting suicide for philosophical reasons (i.e., my life as a schizophrenic is not worth living) is unacceptable and negligent. You must first search for treatable mental states that can drive suicidality, such as depression and demoralization, and you must try to modify a diathesis that makes people suicide-prone. From my point of view as a physician, suicide is not the logical consequence of schizophrenia but the ultimate sad and tragic outcome.

I started this chapter with a quote by Albert Camus. He would surely argue that suicidal thinking cannot be reduced to the clinical concept of "depression," but that a broader frame of reference is required. You will hear this view echoed when patients ask you: "Wouldn't you be depressed and suicidal if you had been told you had schizophrenia?" In essence, your patient is asking, "Is this life still worth living?" Such a question carries the unspoken assumption that nobody can help, particularly not with medicine. Suicide is seen as logical for philosophical reasons; more factors seem to speak for suicide than against it.

I agree with Camus that existential questions matter. After all, medicine is in the business of the human condition with its plights of disease and death. However, we should not accept as the final word the fallacious "balance sheet" thinking of a patient with schizophrenia who has given up. Instead, our therapeutic goal when faced with such demoralized patients is to give back to the patient a vision of his or her future. In Victor Frankl's words, while we often cannot change a situation, we can always choose our attitude toward a situation. As a clinician, this is our responsibility toward suicidal patients: to alleviate suffering that stems from diagnosable, clinical mental states that can lead to suicide. Sometimes medication can alleviate suffering directly by treating positive symptoms or clinical depression or the neurobiology of the suicidal drive. At other times we guide patients psychotherapeutically and we treat demoralization with hope. Suffice it to say, providing longitudinal care and support and accompanying patients through their illness, thereby imbuing patients with a sense of therapeutic optimism, constitute a necessary first step. While not all diseases are curable, all diseases are treatable.

CLINICAL VIGNETTE

Heinz was a 19-year-old young man who had excelled in high school and had gained acceptance into a prestigious college in Cambridge, Massachusetts. A few months into his first semester, he was seen at the student mental health clinic for depression, when he had become withdrawn and stopped going to classes.

A few weeks later, he was admitted to a private hospital in the outskirts of Boston with florid psychosis in the form of paranoia, hallucinations, and disorganized thinking, suggesting that his diagnosis was first-episode schizophrenia. His positive symptoms remitted completely, but his improvement plateaued otherwise and he was unable to return to his school because of subtle cognitive problems and negative symptoms. Three months after his psychotic episode, he took an overdose of over-the-counter sleeping pills.

This patient was at high risk for suicide when he came to understand that schizophrenia might prevent him from pursuing the career he had envisioned. He represents a typical face behind the statistic of 50% lifetime suicide attempts in schizophrenia: he was young, diagnosed with schizophrenia, and he had excellent academic prospects.

ADDITIONAL RESOURCES

Web Sites

http://www.ucalgary.ca/cdss/—The CDSS is available at this Web site. The University of Calgary has a very active schizophrenia research program, and the CDSS comes out of its Department of Psychiatry.

http://www.suicidology.org/—The Web site of the American Association of Suicidology. A good starting point for more information. This site has a large number of links to other organizations and resources related to suicide.

Illness Insight and Medication Adherence

Essential Concepts
- Insight into illness is neither necessary nor sufficient for adherence to medications.
- Illness insight is not a simple, all-or-nothing concept, but is dimensional: awareness of symptoms, acknowledgment of illness, and acceptance of need for treatment.
- Some patients have an anosognosia-like deficit in recognizing that they are psychiatrically ill and could benefit from treatment.
- To assess medication adherence, assess financial barriers, cognitive problems, and health beliefs (which involves a weighing of perceived risks and benefits from the patient's viewpoint).
- Effectiveness of a medicine is driven by its efficacy; nobody likes to take ineffective or marginally effective medications with many side effects.

"The desire to take medicine is perhaps the greatest feature which distinguishes man from animals."
—*Sir William Osler, Father of Modern Medicine, 1849–1919*

"Everything should be made as simple as possible, but not simpler."
—*Albert Einstein*

Adherence to antipsychotics is one of the most important determinants of prognosis in schizophrenia. Recognizing medication adherence problems and identifying reasons for nonadherence are therefore important considerations in the treatment of patients with schizophrenia. Note that "adherence" is now generally preferred over the older, more paternalistic term "compliance."

Families frequently ask for "more therapy" for a nonadherent family member, revealing two assumptions about insight and adherence: (a) that insight is necessary and sufficient for adherence, and (b) that insight is a function of the amount of treatment provided (and hence can increase if enough treatment is given). Unfortunately, insight does not necessarily translate into adherence; and lack of insight sides comfortably with excellent adherence.

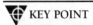 KEY POINT

"Lack of insight" poses one of the biggest obstacles to the treatment of schizophrenia. However, the reverse is not correct: a good understanding of one's illness and the proposed treatment is neither necessary nor sufficient for anyone to take medications.

INSIGHT INTO ILLNESS

In a seminal World Health Organization (WHO) study of schizophrenia, a key finding was that "lack of insight" was the most useful clinical feature in distinguishing schizophrenia from other mental disorders. Consequently, much work has been dedicated to better understand the nature of this lack of insight. Clearly, insight into illness is not the simple shorthand "patient has no insight" that psychiatrists sometimes use to describe patients, particularly patients who disagree with treatment recommendations. Some patients might very well agree with you that they suffer from a mental illness and that they have symptoms, but they do not see medications as the solution. The acceptance of need for treatment, in particular, is shaped by cultural expectations.

The most eloquent, clinical definition of "insight" comes from Sir Aubrey Lewis. He defined insight as "a correct attitude toward a morbid change in oneself." More recent work has stressed that insight is best regarded as a multidimensional construct (David, 1990):

- Awareness of symptoms—Ability to recognize inner experiences or observations as abnormal
- Acknowledgment of illness—Ability to see oneself as suffering from an illness.
- Acceptance of need for treatment—Ability to acknowledge that treatment could be useful, particularly to prevent relapse

TIP

To assess insight as it relates to taking antipsychotics, I focus on acknowledgment of illness and need for treatment: "Do you have any mental health problems? Do you need any treatment for mental health problems? Do your medications do you any good?" (Adapted from the Insight into Treatment Attitude Questionnaire, or ITAQ, developed by Dr. Joseph McEvoy; McEvoy et al., 1989.)

An important question is whether you can improve insight into illness. Some would say that psychosis (particularly delusions) by definition has an element of lack of insight built into the definition. However, patients who are just relapsing or patients in the prodrome of schizophrenia are often able to recognize that something is wrong (abnormal perceptions or attenuated psychosis) and seem to have at least partial insight. This capacity to self-observe and reflect gets lost once patients develop full-blown psychosis or mania. One observation that has been made is that depression adds to the ability to have insight, akin to pain as a warning that something is wrong (Freudenreich et al., 2004a). That said, there are probably some patients who are fundamentally unable to see their symptoms as such. This inability to recognize themselves as somebody with symptoms (suggesting an illness) has been compared to the anosognosia of neurology. Some studies suggest that this aspect of illness is a true neuropsychiatric deficit (Aleman et al., 2006) that you would not expect to be remedied by talking. However, in some patients, "denial" as a psychologic mechanism is probably operative (Cooke et al., 2005), where ongoing conversation can lead to improved insight.

MEDICATION ADHERENCE

Many patients are in fact not "noncompliant" with all aspects of treatment. I treat patients who see me regularly for their appointments but just do not want to take antipsychotics. Others miss their appointments regularly but always call on time to have their medications refilled by the pharmacy. Thus, be clear what you mean if you describe somebody as "noncompliant."

TABLE 29.1. Factors That Contribute to Poor Adherence

Poor symptom control[a]
Medication side effects
Complicated medication regimen
Impaired judgment and insight
Substance use
Real-life, pragmatic problems (money, transportation)
Stigma associated with schizophrenia
Poor therapeutic alliance

[a]Poor medication efficacy is a major obstacle to adherence. Patients who perceive benefit from medications are more willing to take them.

Reasons for Poor Medication Adherence

There is only one way to adhere 100% to medications, but 100 reasons for not adhering (Table 29.1).

Often, you will be able to identify one main obstacle to better adherence. I suggest you look at three key determinants of nonadherence: barriers to health care access, cognitive problems, and health belief models (Perkins, 2002).

Health Care Access Problems

Start with the obvious: an important group of patients takes less medication than prescribed, not because of ill will, but because the patients have no money or because they could not get transportation or for a host of other real-life reasons. Health care is simply not the most important of their many pressing needs. It makes no sense to give patients a prescription they cannot afford. Simply ask, "Can you get this prescription filled today?"

Neuropsychiatric and Cognitive Deficits

Cognitive psychologists differentiate between competence and performance: competence is the potential ability to do something; performance refers to the actual behaviors. Competence is the prerequisite for good performance. Hence, make sure that your patient is not too impaired (i.e., has the competence) to actually implement your recommendations. You need to take into account education and ability to think in abstract terms when you explain your plan. Problems in the cognitive realm should become obvious when you ask the patient to repeat your medication plan: "Tell me again, how are you going to take the medications?"

Health Belief Model

 KEY POINT

According to the health belief model, patients weigh the perceived benefits of treatment with the perceived risks and costs of treatment. Note that it is risks, costs, and benefits from the patient's point of view, not yours.

One prediction from the health belief model is that patients will discontinue medications that they perceive as not working, that seem to have too many side effects compared to the benefits, or that are not deemed necessary to begin with. Note that it is the balance of efficacy and side effects, not simply lack of side effects, that determines adherence in this model: patients with cancer risk dying from their treatment, which can have serious side effects, because of the perceived benefit. A second prediction from the health belief model is that a patient's viewpoint can run counter to society's views: a psychotic patient rejects treatment for fear of side effects, even though society can feel compelled to involuntarily treat or confine the patient for reasons of safety.

Assessment of Medication Adherence

First, you must consider the overwhelming odds of some degree of nonadherence in all chronic disorders, medical and psychiatric. Nonadherence and partial adherence are the norm, not the exception. Studies have shown that physicians routinely overestimate how much of their medications patients are taking. There is no gold standard for assessing medication adherence; each method can be subverted, if so desired. I use a combination of the following to estimate adherence in my patients:

- Directly ask patients to estimate their degree of compliance, for example, "Of the last 5 days, how many days have you missed your pills?"
- Call the pharmacy and see if there are obvious gaps in refilling medications.

- Check antipsychotic serum levels.
- Have patient keep medication log and bring in pills for direct count.
- Ask other people about their views of the patient's compliance.

One of the most under-appreciated problems is partial adherence to antipsychotics. Patients might be taking only some of their medications and honestly think they are doing a good job. This can have pernicious consequences since both you and the patient operate under the assumption that the medication is taken but not working. The lower the maintenance dose, the more magnified partial adherence becomes. Typical results of partial adherence are unnecessarily high medication doses and polypharmacy.

 TIP

Do not overlook partial adherence. Consider partial adherence in any patient whose symptoms are poorly controlled. Each visit, estimate adherence by asking: "In the last 5 days, how many pills have you missed?" This question makes it concrete.

Optimizing Medication Adherence

There are some general things that you should do for all your patients to promote medication adherence:

- Most importantly, focus on patient goals; the medication needs to represent something of value to the patient. For concrete thinkers, the benefit can be concrete, such as staying out of the hospital. If patients are unable to identify a reason they should take their medications, they are unlikely to take them.
- Give patients a positive drug experience—put differently, avoid aversive conditioning, for example, acute dystonic reaction, and do not ignore distressing nonpsychotic symptoms.
- Simple regimens are almost always better. Find qd regimens. Avoid confusing dosing regimens (e.g., different doses of the same medicine).
- Using psychoeducation to provide one explanatory model (i.e., your model, which is the biomedical model). Psychoeducation has to be tailored to the patient's education.

Never give up: I follow patients even if they do not take antipsychotics. Some patients need time and your support over many years. Eventually, some come around and will try an antipsychotic. Following them even when nonadherent gives them a sense of regaining some control over their lives and can strengthen the alliance. However, acknowledge when voluntary treatment is not working and involuntary treatment becomes necessary (see next chapter).

ADDITIONAL RESOURCES

Books

Amador XF, David AS, eds. *Insight and psychosis: Awareness of illness in schizophrenia and related disorders*. New York: Oxford University Press; 2004.—Covers all aspects of insight.
Amador XF. *I'm not sick, I don't need help*. Peconic, NY: Vida Press; 2000.—The best book on the topic of refusal of treatment as a result of impaired insight (Amador suggested the anosognosia analogy for lack of insight in schizophrenia).

Article

Cooke MA, Peters ER, Kuipers E, et al. Disease, deficit or denial? Models of poor insight in psychosis. *Acta Psychiatr Scand.* 2005;112:4–17.—A recent review of competing models of poor insight.

Forensic Aspects of Schizophrenia Care

Essential Concepts

- Physicians have obligations not only toward the welfare of their patients but also toward the commonwealth of the citizens in their community. Protecting the public from harm from psychotic patients is such an obligation that is mandated by state laws.
- Involuntary hospitalization and treatment is necessary and allowed for patients with psychosis who are dangerous to others, to themselves, or who are incapacitated to the point that they can no longer take care of themselves.
- Evaluations for capacity to consent to or refuse medical treatment follow the same principles for patients with schizophrenia as for any other patients.
- Lack of appropriate paternalism in health care can result in patient abandonment.

". . . nor shall any State deprive any person of life, liberty, or property, without due process of law."
Fourteenth Amendment to the United States Constitution

A fundamental right in our society is that citizens have the "right to be let alone," in Supreme Court Justice Louis Brandeis's words. In the medical arena, this means that (competent) patients can refuse even life saving treatments. However, the public also has the right to be protected, and physicians have obligations toward the welfare of the general public as well. In disorders that potentially affect a community, the personal perspective is important but not sufficient to ignore community interests. Just as patients might not have the right go untreated and spread tuberculosis, they might not have the right to endanger other people while psychotic.

TIP

Be a good clinician, not a bad lawyer: provide good clinical care based on respect for patient autonomy but also based on the values of nonmaleficence and beneficence. Do not give bad legal advice, but consult a lawyer for legal questions. Obviously, know and follow the laws of the land as they pertain to your practice.

VIOLENCE

A link between psychosis and violence has been much debated and at times even discounted, probably because of efforts to decrease stigma. I think it defies common sense that psychosis would not in certain instances increase the risk for violence: it obviously does. The most dangerous patients I have encountered come from a small subgroup of persons with schizophrenia: young, substance-using male patients who are antisocial, and suffer from paranoid schizophrenia. When decompensated, these patients are extremely volatile and paranoid, with no impulse control, which makes them dangerous.

 TIP

The most useful predictors of violence are any past history of violence and substance use. Therefore, get a good legal history, previous arrests, prison time, and exact legal charges. Go back to middle school and look for a conduct disorder and early substance use.

The Clinical Antipsychotic Trials of Intervention Effectiveness (CATIE) evaluated the propensity for violence in their sample of almost 1,500 patients. The 6-month prevalence for any act of violence was close to 20% (Swanson et al., 2006). You should note, however, that serious violence (in this study defined as assault resulting in injury, lethal weapon threat or use, or sexual assault) was much less common, 3.6%. Serious violence was associated with positive symptoms, whereas other forms of violence were better predicted by environmental variables. Not surprisingly, negative symptoms had a protective effect.

TIP

It is not psychosis per se that determines the risk of violence but the nature of the delusion (particularly thoughts of persecution) and hallucinations (i.e., command type). Find out exactly what patients are thinking and engage them in a discussion of violence, for example, how likely they think it is that they will take preventive or retaliatory action.

You must know your legal responsibilities with regard to warning identified victims and protecting them and the public (the so-called duty to warn and protect). To safeguard the public, all states have provisions for committing a patient with schizophrenia who is violent.

Here are some key points to remember to stay safe in your line of work as a psychiatrist treating schizophrenia:

- When you work with psychotic patients, remain alert to the possibility of harm from your patient.
- Just like you assess the potential for suicide in all patients, you must estimate the risk for immediate violence and the potential for violence in the future. You do this by combining an actuarial approach (past history) with your cross-sectional data (Table 30.1).
- Record any history of violence during acute psychosis in your lifetime problem list so the information does not get lost.

Preventing violence is important not just to protect yourself and society but also to combat stigma. Allowing a small

TABLE 30.1. Clinical Assessment of Aggression[a]

Excitement	Is the patient motorically accelerated and pressured in his or her speech (this looks hypomanic)?
Hostility	Is the patient angry and irritable? Sarcastic? Resentful?
Uncooperativeness	Does the patient refuse to comply with tasks asked of him or her?
Poor impulse control	How well is the patient able to tolerate frustration? Does the patient fly off the handle regardless of consequences?

[a]These four items are taken from the Positive and Negative Syndrome Scale (PANSS), in which they comprise the Excited Cluster.

subset of violent persons with schizophrenia to go untreated is a disservice to all patients with schizophrenia who are trying to live peaceful lives.

The most effective interventions to prevent more violence from high-risk patients target these three areas:

- Nonadherence—Consider long-acting antipsychotics. Refer to ACT teams (Table 30.2), if available. Consider outpatient commitments if available.
- Drug use—In some jurisdictions, probation and court-mandated treatment (e.g., random urine drug testing) instead of prison time can provide motivation. In some programs, entitlement benefits can be contingent on drug-free status.
- Residual psychosis—Use the most effective antipsychotics, including clozapine; clozapine also has antiaggressive properties independent of its antipsychotic properties.

INVOLUNTARY TREATMENT

Prior to the 1960s, involuntary civil commitments were largely left to the discretion of psychiatrists if there seemed to be a "need for treatment." With the rise of the civil liberties movement, this prerogative has been severely curtailed, and patients today are committed for "danger to self or others" and no longer for need for treatment. Many think the pendulum has swung too far and rightly point to the difficulties in getting psychotic but nondangerous patients appropriately treated if they refuse treatment. A purely rights-based approach that includes the right to refuse treatment negates the clinical reality of an anosognosia-like inability to see oneself as ill and in need of treatment.

◆ KEY POINT

Currently, the threshold for involuntary intervention is high, usually dangerousness to self or others or clear inability to care for oneself. The dangerousness or inability to care for oneself must stem from a mental illness. Psychiatric (civil) commitment is usually a two-step process; the initial involuntary hospitalization, which can be initiated by a physician, and a petition to the court for psychiatric commitment, which may or may not be granted. Technically, it is not psychiatrists but judges who "commit" patients, a point often overlooked. State laws vary considerably on the details.

I view an involuntary hospitalization and treatment as the gateway to eventual voluntary treatment and as a tool to restore capacity lost during psychosis. These are the three typical clinical situations in which you should seek involuntary hospitalization and treatment for psychotic patients who refuse treatment:

- Potentially violent patients, to reduce risk to specific people or the community at large. This is the typical case of commitment for "danger to others" and refers to dangerousness due to symptoms of a psychiatric illness. You act as an agent of the state to protect the community, but you also act as the patient's advocate to protect the patient from legal charges and criminalization or injury.
- Psychotic patient at acute risk for a suicide attempt. This is the case of commitment for "danger to self."
- Patients who are unable to care for themselves while psychotic. This is the remnant of the in-need-for-treatment approach. Depending on the exact interpretation and wording of the respective statute, this can be very difficult to apply, and judges might have a threshold very different from yours. Are you unable to care for yourself if you can line up in a shelter line and find the local soup kitchen?

CLINICAL VIGNETTE

Franz was a promising college student who developed persecutory delusions and left college. Despite attempts to initiate treatment with an antipsychotic, he resisted as he was convinced that there was "nothing wrong" with him. An involuntary hospitalization was initiated, but the petition for civil commitment was not granted, as Franz was eloquent in the hearing and had neither been homeless, without food (he had moved back in with his parents), nor dangerous. Months later, a second treatment attempt, after some admittedly vague threats, led to a period of involuntary hospitalization "for dangerousness" and treatment, leading to full recovery.

This patient represents a subgroup of patients who fall through the cracks: clearly psychotic, yet resisting any treatment; at the same time, not clearly dangerous (but also not doing well, with their lives wrecked by decisions made under the influence of delusions). Often, the outcome of a hearing depends on the judge's view of mental illness and its treatments. Families might have little leverage in compelling such "quietly psychotic" family members to begin treatment, short of evicting their family member or withdrawing resources. In this case, the patient was grateful for the episode of involuntary treatment, after he had recovered (some remain furious).

Sometimes you are asked (by the group home, the family, or the police) to simply hospitalize somebody because of some potential for violence sometime in the future. It is not your task as a physician to prevent commission of violence by antisocial or angry people; your role is to treat patients who are dangerous because of psychiatric illness. Be wary of colluding with anything that would more aptly be termed preventive detention. Preventive detention and involuntary confinement (without treatment) are police functions.

States continue to experiment with legislation and treatment models that entail an element of coercion. The availability of assisted treatment options short of involuntary hospitalizations varies greatly by state or even county (Table 30.2).

TABLE 30.2. Assisted Treatment Options for Psychotic Disorders

Advanced (psychiatric) directives	A document put together while well that specifies treatment preferences when ill
Outpatient commitment	Patients are ordered by a court to comply with treatment to be allowed to stay in the community
Conditional-release arrangement	Patients are released from the hospital under the promise of compliance
Assertive community treatment	A well-studied model of care in which patients are tracked down in the community if they miss appointments; this model of case management linked closely with treatment is most effective in reducing hospitalizations and became necessary during the period of deinstitutionalization
Representative payee	Benefit payments are not given directly to patients but are used as incentives to adhere to treatment

CAPACITY EVALUATIONS

Psychiatrists typically are asked to evaluate patients with schizophrenia for "competence" if patients refuse a medical intervention deemed necessary by a physician. Sometimes all that is needed is spending a little more time to explain the risks and benefits to the patient. Evaluations of capacity to make medical decisions follow the same principles for patients with schizophrenia as for other patients. Psychotic patients cannot be considered incompetent merely by virtue of their diagnosis, or in the words of one patient, "I might have schizophrenia but I am not stupid." Make sure, however, that psychosis is not responsible for treatment refusal. Other areas of dysfunction, for example, negative symptoms or cognitive problems, are as important to assess as positive symptoms. Also, as with other patients, you are not trying to assess some "global" capacity, but capacity with regard to a very specific clinical question.

 TIP

The most useful question to ask yourself is this one: "Does the patient appreciate the pragmatic consequences downstream of placing an act now (Phrase courtesy of George B. Murray, MD)." In other words, does the patient truly appreciate what it means tomorrow if he refuses to have surgery today? The key word is appreciation, in contradistinction to lip service. Patients with clinically relevant executive dysfunction will invariably fail this question.

If patients are unable to recognize that they are ill, guardianship should be considered because such patients are unable to provide meaningful informed consent to treatment. Lip service assenting to treatment is not informed consent. Patients under guardianship often benefit from the additional oversight and help with decisions, allowing them to live in the community.

PATERNALISM IN HEALTH CARE

Paternalism has gotten a bad reputation as it seemingly conflicts with patient autonomy. However, patient autonomy can be impaired by poor judgment, and focusing solely on autonomy ignores the obvious fact that physicians, as experts with experience, sometimes do know better, and that patients make bad decisions that run counter to their own long-term interests. Physicians have always provided guidance (i.e., paternalism), and paternalism has always been constrained by the time-honored principles of nonmaleficence and benevolence. Helping patients make good decisions can be an intrusion into their lives. However, if seen as a tool to advance true autonomy, patients ultimately benefit. Insisting on a representative payee to manage benefit payments is an example of paternalism. True, the patient can no longer choose to spend the money on drugs and alcohol, and will not sleep in a shelter because of lack of rent payment. However, help with money can be the first step toward more responsible budgeting and, ultimately, secure housing. What exactly is respected if your psychotic patients languish in a homeless shelter, their civil rights seemingly intact?

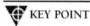 KEY POINT

Not pursuing assisted treatment options out of undue respect for autonomy can be a form of abandonment and ignores the equally important principles of nonmaleficence and benevolence. A lack of appropriate paternalism does not respect patient autonomy. The consequences of no treatment are victimization, homelessness, criminalization, or abandoned careers, to suggest a few.

ADDITIONAL RESOURCES

Web Sites

http://www.psychlaws.org—The Treatment Advocacy Center (TAC) Web site; TAC advocates for better involuntary treatment options for vulnerable populations, as opposed to letting patients go untreated. The Web site also has a list of state laws relevant to assisted treatment.

Books

Earley P. *Crazy: A father's search through America's mental health madness.* New York: G. P. Putnam's Sons; 2006.— Earley, journalist and father, chronicles the sad story of his son with mental illness, as both move through the American legal system. After reading the book, you will appreciate the shortcomings of our current approach to refusal of treatment for mental illness.

31

Social Aspects of Schizophrenia Care

Essential Concepts

- You cannot practice medicine without considering the impact of societal factors like poverty or homelessness on illness.
- Patients with a stigmatizing illness like schizophrenia suffer from both the illness *and the reaction of people to the illness.*
- The current mental health care system is unable to provide the lifelong, high-quality services that patients with schizophrenia need to function optimally.

"Truly I say to you, to the extent that you did it to one of these brothers of Mine, even the least of them, you did it to Me."
—*Matthew 25:40 (New American Standard Bible)*

A useful distinction can be made between the sociology *in* psychiatry and the sociology *of* psychiatry. The sociology *in* psychiatry concerns itself with the impact (either causative or modifying) of social factors on disease (e.g., the role of anomie in suicide, the role of immigration on schizophrenia risk, the role of family stress on relapse risk, the effects of class and race on health). The sociology *of* psychiatry examines psychiatry's role in societies, particularly with regard to social control of "deviance" (e.g., the effects of getting a stigmatizing disease label; the parameters for involuntary treatment; the function of the state hospital as a "total institution," a term coined by Erving Goffman). Many sociologic aspects of care are discussed throughout this book. In this chapter, I focus on social adversity, stigma, and the current health care system.

SOCIAL ADVERSITY

 KEY POINT

A problem without a solution is not a need for psychiatry.*
However, many intractable social problems like poverty and
homelessness are exactly the problems that your patients
struggle with and that have an impact on prognosis.

It is impossible to practice medicine without acknowledging the
social realities of patients. Paul Farmer, an infectious disease
specialist who has spent most of his career traveling between
Harvard and Haiti to bring modern medicine to rural Haiti, has
stressed the importance of biosocial causation of illnesses. It is
not possible to isolate an illness and study its "natural course"
without considering how people ended up in harm's way, their
access to care, and their adherence to treatment. Farmer uses
the term "structural violence" (a term coined by Johan Galtung
and by liberation theologians in the 1960s to denote social
structures that impede humans from reaching their potential) to
emphasize the pernicious effects of adverse social conditions on
clinical outcomes. The "natural" history of tuberculosis varies
greatly, depending on where and how you contract the
bacterium and what kind of treatment you get. Similarly, the
"natural" history of schizophrenia will be difficult to understand if social factors are ignored.

The social consequences of schizophrenia are rather significant. Having schizophrenia puts you at an economic disad-
vantage, and many patients experience a downward social
drift into unemployment and poverty (social selection theory). A significant minority of the homeless population has
schizophrenia, perhaps as many as 15% to 30%, probably for
the most part due to lack of affordable housing.

 TIP

Bad economic conditions (in other words, poverty) are real
for many of your patients. Try to understand the barriers that
poverty or living in a shelter puts up for each patient, particularly with regard to adherence.

*Attributed to Norman Sartorius during Grand Rounds at Cambridge Hospital, Cambridge,
Massachusetts, in 2006.

STIGMA

It is a myth that "schizophrenia is an illness like any other." If it were, patients would not have to decide whom they are going to tell about it. Schizophrenia is a highly stigmatizing condition; being afflicted with it leaves the sufferer with a "mark or token of infamy, disgrace or reproach." Stigma is a powerful psychologic force and a societal reality for patients with mental disorders, including schizophrenia. The pervasive emotion attached to stigma is shame, leading patients to deny illness, hide symptoms from others, and refuse to seek care. Shame can be pervasive in families themselves; you can see this in families in which a positive family history of psychotic illness might never be acknowledged.

🌐 KEY POINT

Schizophrenia is not "an illness like any other." In contrast to other illnesses, patients with stigmatizing illnesses like schizophrenia have to face the disease itself and their own and society's reactions to having the disease. Reactions include shame on the inside with reluctance to seek help, and prejudice and rejection outside with social exclusion.

Stigma leads to social exclusion from full community participation and loss of opportunity. Unemployment is but one form of social exclusion, and patients often do not vote, do not go to church anymore, etc. A vicious cycle is set into motion since unemployment leads to poverty, which limits opportunities that we take for granted (e.g., a vacation). Subtle forms of exclusion can be seen in discriminating practices and legislation, e.g., lack of parity between medical and psychiatric care. Patients also contribute to stigma through internalization of the prevailing cultural stereotypes of mental illness. This attitude is disastrous since patients will give up even trying to build a new life. The resulting social isolation is a form of psychologic death (and can precipitate suicide).

Psychiatry, while well intentioned, inadvertently contributed to stigma by insisting on a "broken brain" model of mental illness and placing less emphasis on psychosocial determinants. Patients and the public clearly prefer psychosocial explanations as a more hopeful model since it allows for (self-) control. Particularly in first-episode patients, a more sophisticated view of psychosis that allows for societal factors seems to be more useful. Another area in which psychiatry contributed to stigma was by propagating that patients with mental illness are not more dangerous than the general population. Nothing stigmatizes more patients with mental illness than the one, highly publicized case in which a patient who was allowed to go untreated pushed somebody in front of a subway.

The consequences of stigma for patients are real, and many patients struggle with these questions at some point during their illness or even their whole lives:

- The issue of disclosure: Who, what, and when should I tell about my mental illness? How do I explain a gap in my resume caused by being hospitalized?
- How are my friends going to view me? Am I still worthy?
- The issue of self-blame: What did I do wrong?
- Is it true, I have a mental illness? How should I conceptualize schizophrenia? Which model of causation of mental illness should I adopt (biogenetic versus psychosocial)?
- How can I get integrated into a society that values work so much, even if I do not work?
- Is my life worth living?

As a way of decreasing stigma, some have suggested changing the name of schizophrenia to, say, Kraepelin's disease. I am unsure if that would really make a difference. I find Susan Sontag's argument better, that schizophrenia will cease to be stigmatizing once it ceases to be a metaphor (in this case, for unpredictability and lack of control).

 TIP

It is important to recall the images that "schizophrenia" conjures up in nonexperts, and accordingly be very cautious about how you introduce the idea of schizophrenia and how you talk about it. Do not avoid the term but be cognizant of its associations and be flexible in working with how patients see causation.

When patients first get ill, they and their families know as much about schizophrenia as the general public: very little. Most would be hard-pressed to explain the difference between multiple personalities, psychopathy, and schizophrenia; or to identify hallucinations as a core feature. Many would probably equate schizophrenia with unpredictable violence. Psychoeducation of patients and families and referral to reputable sources are important ways to help patients and their families overcome stereotypes of schizophrenia (see Chapter 18).

MENTAL HEALTH CARE TREATMENT SYSTEM

Any health care system is the result of large historical and societal forces, and I conclude this book with a brief section on our mental health care system since the availability and affordability of services will have an impact on any clinical decision that you make.

History of Schizophrenia Care in the United States

Schizophrenia is a young disease, first described in its current, recognizable form by Emil Kraepelin in 1893, little more than 100 years ago. Named dementia praecox by Kraepelin, Eugen Bleuler gave schizophrenia its current name. The basic concept of schizophrenia as a nonepisodic psychiatric illness characterized by the predominance of typical symptoms of psychosis has not changed much since these early pioneers described this disease entity. What has changed is the way we treat schizophrenia. In Kraepelin's days, psychiatrists (or rather "alienists," as they were called) practiced in state hospitals. Most patients with schizophrenia, once admitted to a state hospital, would live out their natural lives in these total institutions (a term the anthropologist Irving Goffman uses to describe settings where people are taken care of in their totality, e.g., prisons or the military).

Today, most patients are cared for in the community. This is the result of medical progress (chlorpromazine became widely available for clinical use in 1954) and legislation (President John F. Kennedy signed the Community Mental Health Centers Act in 1963), which together allowed for the emptying of state hospitals, known as deinstitutionalization. Some have argued that we did not have deinstitutionalization in the United States but "dehospitalization," with most people who used to be institutionalized in state institutions now at best "institutionalized in the community," or worse "transinstitutionalized" into jails and prisons, or homeless. An interesting proposition is that each society tolerates a certain, fixed amount of deviancy or pathology; whether a deviant person is dealt with through the penal system or the medical system depends only on the availability of beds. If psychiatric beds are scarce, rather than being brought to a hospital, patients are arrested and diverted into the criminal justice system, a phenomenon known as "criminalization of the mentally ill."

I also like to point out the diametrically opposed associations that people have when they conjure up images of an "asylum" or the "community." It should not be forgotten that state hospitals were once seen as "asylums," as places from which vulnerable people could not be expelled, as one meaning of asylum. This view of asylum changed when what once was a good idea was turned upside down by overcrowding. Conversely, while "community" conjures up images of peace and happiness, patients can be institutionalized in the community in the middle of downtown Boston, not partaking in civic life but wasting away in poorly run group homes, with little to no interaction with the community at large. A small subgroup of very vulnerable patients no longer has the option of living in an asylum.

The Current U.S. Nonsystem of Care

The promises and hopes of deinstitutionalization never materialized. As anyone treating the typical ambulatory patient with schizophrenia will discover quickly, high-quality services beyond acute care beds are simply not widely available, and patients often receive little more than medications. Those rehabilitation services that exist are often underfunded and poorly staffed. Too often, you succeed for brief periods not because of the support of a comprehensive treatment system but because of your persistence and individual, random acts of kindness, for example, an insurance person extending a direly needed hospital stay for another 3 days. Sadly, dedication alone, without financial support and a larger system of care to back you up, seems to be the current American solution for mental health.

I am going to end this book with an inspiration and obligation found as an inscription on a fountain in Cambridge, Massachusetts. These are the words of President John Fitzgerald Kennedy from his Address to the Massachusetts Legislature 11 days before his inauguration, on January 9, 1961:

> *When at some future date the high court of history sits in*
> *judgment on each of us . . . our success or failure in whatever*
> *office we hold will be measured by the answers to four questions:*

> *Were we truly men of courage . . .? Were we truly men of integrity . . .?*
> *Were we truly men of judgment . . .? Were we truly men of dedication . . .?*

> *The enduring qualities of Massachusetts—*
> *the common threads woven by the Pilgrim and the Puritan,*
> *the fisherman and the farmer, the Yankee and the immigrant—*
> *are an indelible part of my life, my convictions,*
> *my view of the past, and my hopes for the future.*

ADDITIONAL RESOURCES

Book

Whitaker R. *Mad in America: Bad science, bad medicine, and the enduring mistreatment of the mentally ill.* Cambridge, MA: Perseus; 2002.—Written for the lay public by a journalist, a controversial, sometimes inaccurate but always engaging critical view of psychiatric care over three centuries. Take it with a grain of salt but do not dismiss it summarily.

Article

Weissman MM. Stigma [A piece of my mind]. *JAMA.* 2001;285:261–262.—If you believe there is parity between medical care and mental health care, read this essay about one patient and his mother who encounter both treatment systems.

APPENDICES

Emergency Cards

EM CARD ACUTE BEHAVIORAL DISTURBANCE

The following medications are options for acutely agitated, healthy adult patients who need immediate treatment of agitation in an emergency department setting. Choice and suggested doses need to be modified based on the clinical situation.

First-Line Options

If patient accepts oral medication:

- Diazepam 5 to 10 mg po.[a] Can repeat twice after 30 to 60 minutes.
- Lorazepam 1 to 2 mg po/sublingual. Can repeat twice after 30 to 60 minutes.
- Olanzapine 10 to 15 mg po. Can repeat after 1 hour. Available as orally disintegrating tablet (ODT). Note that ODTs are not absorbed by the oral mucosa: They must still be swallowed!
- Risperidone 1 to 2 mg. Can repeat after 1 hour. Available as liquid and ODT.

If patient refuses oral medication:

- Lorazepam 1 to 2 mg intramuscularly (IM). Can repeat every 20 minutes.[b]
- Haloperidol 5 to 10 mg plus lorazepam 2 mg plus benztropine 1 mg IM.[b]
- Haloperidol 5 to 10 mg plus lorazepam 2 mg plus diphenhydramine 50 mg IM.[b]
- Olanzapine 10 mg IM. Can repeat in 2 hours; up to three doses/day.
- Ziprasidone 20 mg IM. Can repeat in 4 hours; up to two doses/day. Monitor QTc.

---

[a]Oral onset almost as fast as IV onset. Do not give IM because of erratic absorption.

[b]Repeat every 20 minutes if no effect. Once haloperidol 20 mg TDD is given, use only benzodiazepines. Give only two doses of benztropine/diphenhydramine per 24 hours (anticholinergic delirium). Use higher doses of lorazepam (e.g., more than 6 mg) only in settings where flumazenil and ventilation are available.

Second-Line Options

- Chlorpromazine 50 to 100 mg IM (CAVE never IV: hypotension; IM more potent than po).
- Aripiprazole is available as oral solution, ODT, and IM injection (9.75 mg) for emergency use; clinical experience is limited.
- Benzodiazepines can be given IV by slow bolus injection,[c] e.g., lorazepam, diazepam, midazolam.
- Haloperidol can also be given IV or by drip.[d]

[c]Use only in settings where flumazenil is available and ventilation is possible.
[d]Use only in settings with cardiac monitoring, monitor the QTc and replete potassium and magnesium to decrease risk of torsades de pointes. (see EM CARD IV Haloperidol).

EM CARD IV HALOPERIDOL (HALDOL)

- Treatment of acute agitation: Goal is calm, but awake.
- Start by ensuring an adequate medical workup and optimize medical management:
  1. Check ECG: If QTc >450, consider alternatives. Always check the QTc manually, as the machine-calculated QTc is prone to error. The formula is QTc = QT divided by (R-R interval)exp1/2.
  2. Check Mg (replete to Mg $\geq$2). Check K (replete to K $\geq$4).
  3. Haldol 5 mg^e IV $\times$ 1, wait 20 to 30 minutes.
  4. If still agitated in 20 to 30 minutes, recheck ECG. If QTc >450 or increased by 25%, consider alternatives or consult cardiology and use telemetry.
  5. Double (or repeat) Haldol dosage, and go back to step 4.^{f}
  6. Once no longer agitated, give the final dose as a divided dose over the next 24 hours.
  7. If patient remains calm, reduce dose by 50% every 24 hours and discontinue haloperidol as soon as possible.

Example

Haldol 5 $\rightarrow$ still agitated after 30 minutes $\rightarrow$ Haldol 10 mg $\rightarrow$ still agitated after 30 minutes $\rightarrow$ Haldol 20 mg $\rightarrow$ calm, awake after 30 minutes. Then give Haldol 5 mg IV q6hrs $\times$ 24 hours (for total of 20 mg).

Notes

- Keep in mind that Haldol precipitates with *heparin and phenytoin* and should not be administered in the same line.
- Oral haloperidol dose is twice the IV dose.
- If Haldol causes adverse reaction, including prolonged QTc, consider alternatives: Zyprexa (olanzapine) 5 to 10 mg, Risperdal (risperidone) 1 to 2 mg, Seroquel (quetiapine) 12.5 to 50 mg, benzodiazepines (but watch for worsening confusion or disinhibition).

(Modified after MGH/McLean Resident Training Handbook.)

---

^{e}For mild agitation 0.5 to 2 mg, for moderate agitation 2 to 5 mg, for severe agitation 5 to 10 mg; if patients are frail or antipsychotic-naïve, start with 0.5 to 2 mg regardless of level of agitation.
^{f}If no response after three doses, add or alternate with lorazepam 0.5 to 1 mg IV.

EM CARD SUICIDE ASSESSMENT

The ABCs of suicide:

A Acute assessment (acute medical concerns)
B Behavioral dissection (facts and chronology)
C Crisis
D Diagnostic 4 Ds (depressed, deranged, disturbed, delirious/diseased)
E Ethanol and drugs
F Family (and personal) history of suicide
G Gun availability
H Homicide risk
I Infanticide risk

(Adapted from Freudenreich O, *J Clin Psychiatry.* 2005;66: 1194–1195.)

Brief instructions for use:

- Make sure you address acute medical concerns after a suicide attempt (e.g., cardiac monitoring).
- Behavioral dissection is an interviewing technique that will help you get down to the facts and chronology, instead of relying on vagueness and opinion, to determine exactly what happened. You basically keep asking: "And then, what exactly did you do?" And you press for details: "Did you put the gun in your mouth or just hold it in your lap?"
- Understand the crisis that pushed the patient over the edge. A crisis is often a loss, which can be the loss of an idea or the [patient's] future.
- Rule out four treatable diagnoses that increase suicide risk. Of the diagnostic 4 Ds (depressed; deranged, as in a psychotic state; disturbed, as in personality disordered; and delirious/diseased, as in suffering from a medical illness), depression and psychosis are the two most important psychiatric conditions that need to be diagnosed and optimally treated.
- The remaining elements of the ABCs are self-explanatory and can serve as a checklist to make sure that you do not overlook other important considerations.

Notes

- Use "The ABCs of suicide" to comprehensively review important clinical data that go into the suicide risk assessment.

- The ABCs are based on the Mann et al. stress-diathesis model to understand suicidality and help you collect the facts about a suicide attempt or suicidal ideation, the proximate events leading to a suicidal crisis, and the distal diathesis that might put somebody at higher suicide risk to begin with.

ADDITIONAL RESOURCES

Freudenreich O. The ABCs of suicide [letter]. *J Clin Psychiatry.* 2005;66:1194–1195.—I explain in more detail the rationale and the use of the "ABCs" to assess suicidality.

Assessment Scale Cards

SCALE CARD ABNORMAL INVOLUNTARY MOVEMENT SCALE (AIMS)

The AIMS is a well-established rating scale for involuntary movements during antipsychotic treatment; it can be used to comprehensively assess a patient for movements typical for tardive dyskinesia and to rate their severity, if present.

Use a 5-point rating scale to rate the severity of items:

0. None (normal)
1. Minimal (maybe extreme normal); use if unsure if abnormal
2. Mild; use if obviously abnormal to a trained observer
3. Moderate; use if layperson would notice
4. Severe

Using the above scale, rate abnormal movements separately for seven body areas (grouped into three bigger areas):

Facial and oral movements

1. Muscles of facial expression (e.g., frowning, blinking, grimacing)
2. Lips and perioral area (e.g., puckering, pouting, smacking)
3. Jaw (e.g., biting, clenching, chewing, mouth opening, lateral movements)
4. Tongue (i.e., increase in movement in and out of mouth)

Extremity movements

5. Upper extremity
6. Lower extremity (e.g., foot tapping, squirming, inversion or eversion)

Trunk movements

7. Neck, shoulder, hips (e.g., rocking, twisting, squirming, pelvic gyrations)

Create two severity scores:

AIMS total score: add up items 1 to 7 (often used in research)
Overall severity score: use the 5-point scale to estimate overall severity of abnormal movements

Notes

- The AIMS should be regarded merely as a checklist that allows you to monitor (and record) the severity of involuntary movements. It is not a diagnostic tool!

- Obviously, make sure that the patient is not chewing gum, or has major problems with ill-fitting dentures that the patient tries to keep in place during the examination.
- It is an interesting observation that patients are often unaware of their movements; ask them if they realize they have these movements.

ADDITIONAL RESOURCES

Guy W. ECDEU assessment manual for psychopharmacology. Rockville, MD: U.S. Department of Health, Education, and Welfare; 1976.—The original reference, which you will have great difficulties getting your hands on.

Web Site

http://www.psychiatrictimes.com/scales/—The AIMS is available as a PDF from this site.

Article

Munetz MR, Benjamin S. How to examine patients using the Abnormal Involuntary Movement Scale. *Hosp Community Psychiatry.* 1988;39:1172–1177.—The standard reference, with clear instructions about how to use the AIMS.

SCALE CARD BRIEF PSYCHIATRIC RATING SCALE (BPRS-18$_{1-7}$)

The Brief Psychiatric Rating Scale (BPRS) is a widely used scale to capture the severity of psychopathology in patients with schizophrenia and other psychiatric disorders.

Use the following 7-point severity scale:

1. Not reported
2. Very mild
3. Mild
4. Moderate
5. Moderately severe
6. Severe
7. Very severe

Rate each of the following items (for past week as timeframe):

1. Somatic concern (concern for physical problems)
2. Anxiety
3. Emotional withdrawal (observed related to interviewer)
4. **Conceptual disorganization**[a] (observed thought disorder)
5. Guilt feelings
6. Tension (observed motor restlessness)
7. Mannerisms and posturing (observed abnormal motor behaviors)
8. Grandiosity
9. Depressive mood
10. Hostility
11. **Suspiciousness**[a]
12. **Hallucinatory behavior**[a] (i.e., hallucinations)
13. Motor retardation (observed)
14. Uncooperativeness
15. **Unusual thought content**[a] (i.e., delusions)
16. Blunted affect
17. Excitement
18. Disorientation

Notes

- The BPRS is filled out quickly but has limitations. Negative symptoms are poorly captured; you need to supplement, e.g., with the SANS (see SCALE CARD SANS)

[a]BPRS psychosis cluster.

- There are different versions of the BPRS out there. You should use the 18-item version (not the original 16-item scale, which does not contain excitement and disorientation), with severity rating ranging from 1 to 7 (not 0 to 6).
- Consult the anchored version, BPRS-A, by Woerner et al. (see Additional Resources) to get comfortable with this scale.
- Leucht et al. (see Additional Resources) suggest the following clinical cutoffs for BPRS scores in relation to CGI-S ratings of clinical severity:

Mildly ill	*BPRS 32*
Moderately ill	*BPRS 44*
Markedly ill	*BPRS 55*
Severely ill	*BPRS 70*
Extremely ill	*BPRS 85*

ADDITIONAL RESOURCES

Web sites

http://www.psychiatrictimes.com/scales/—You can download a PDF of the BPRS.

Articles

Leucht S, Kane JM, Kissling W, et al. Clinical implications of Brief Psychiatric Rating Scale scores. *Br J Psychiatry.* 2005; 187:366–371.
Woerner MG, Mannuzza S, Kane JM. Anchoring the BPRS: An aid to improved reliability. *Psychopharmacol Bull.* 1988; 24:112–117.

SCALE CARD GLOBAL ASSESSMENT OF FUNCTIONING (GAF)

Try to put a single number on the patient's mental health, using a scale from 0 to 100. Take into account symptoms, social (interpersonal), and school/occupational (role) functioning, and dangerousness.

91–100	No symptoms Superior function
81–90	No or minimal symptoms Good function
71–80	Transient and expectable symptoms to stressor Slight if any functional impairment
61–70	Mild symptoms Mild social difficulties (e.g., truancy; has friends)
51–60	Moderate symptoms (e.g., panic attacks) Moderate social difficulties (few friends, conflict with co-workers)
41–50	Serious symptoms (e.g., suicidal ideation, obsessive rituals) Serious social difficulties (no friends, cannot keep a job)
31–40	Some psychotic symptoms Major impairment in several areas
21–30	Significant psychotic symptoms or impaired judgment Inability to function in almost all areas (e.g., stays in bed all day)
11–20	Some danger of suicide or violence Difficulties maintaining minimal hygiene Incoherent or mute
0–10	Persistent danger of suicide or violence Persistent inability to maintain minimal hygiene

Notes

- The GAF combines several not necessarily related dimensions of mental health. Choose the domain most severely affected for your rating.

- Note that patients with any (active) psychosis are technically rated as 40 or lower, depending on the severity and functional relevance of their psychotic symptoms.
- Note that dangerous patients are rated as 20 or lower.

(Adapted from the GAF in: American Psychiatric Association. *Diagnostic and statistical manual of mental disorders.* 4th ed., text rev. 2000.)

ADDITIONAL RESOURCES

Article

Goldman HH. Do you walk to school, or do you carry your lunch? [editorial]. *Psychiatr Serv.* 2005;56:419.—Read an editorial in *Psychiatric Services* about the GAF.

SCALE CARD SCALE FOR THE ASSESSMENT OF NEGATIVE SYMPTOMS (SANS)

The Scale for the Assessment of Negative Symptoms was developed to comprehensively rate the negative symptoms of schizophrenia.

Use the following 6-point severity scale:

0. Normal
1. Questionable
2. Mild
3. Moderate
4. Marked
5. Severe

Rate each of the following four items:

1. **Affective flattening or blunting**
   Take into account facial expression, body language, prosody, eye contact, lack of smiling or laughter
2. **Alogia**
   Take into account amount of speech, content of speech, blocking, and latency
3. **Avolition-apathy**
   Take into account grooming and hygiene, impersistence, idleness
4. **Anhedonia-asociality**
   Take into account patient's interest in leisure and relationships

Notes

- Various scoring methods are used for the SANS. You could use the global SANS score by adding up your four ratings (range 0 to 20).
- Like most authors, I skipped "attention," which was a domain in the original scale but which is no longer considered a negative symptom.

ADDITIONAL RESOURCES

Article

Andreasen NC. Negative symptoms in schizophrenia: Definition and reliability. *Arch Gen Psychiatry.* 1982;39:784–788.—The origin of the SANS.

Wellness Cards

WELL CARD BODY MASS INDEX (BMI)

BMI Formula

BMI = weight (in kilogram) divided by height (in meter squared)
BMI = [weight (in pounds) divided by height (in inches squared)]
× 703

Definitions*

BMI range
Normal weight   *18.5 to 24.9*
Overweight   *25 to 29.9*
Obese   *30 to 39.0*
Morbid obesity   *40+*

How to measure waist circumference: Identify upper-most lateral border of iliac crest as bony landmark and measure circumference at that height.

Electronic BMI calculator: http://www.nhlbisupport.com/bmi/

---

*For adults. For children and teenagers, see http://apps.nccd.cdc.gov/dnpabmi/Calculator.aspx.

TABLE C.1 BMI

Body Mass Index Table

	Normal						Overweight					Obese										Extreme Obesity														
BMI	19	20	21	22	23	24	25	26	27	28	29	30	31	32	33	34	35	36	37	38	39	40	41	42	43	44	45	46	47	48	49	50	51	52	53	54
Height (inches)												Body Weight (pounds)																								
58	91	96	100	105	110	115	119	124	129	134	138	143	148	153	158	162	167	172	177	181	186	191	196	201	205	210	215	220	224	229	234	239	244	248	253	258
59	94	99	104	109	114	119	124	128	133	138	143	148	153	158	163	168	173	178	183	188	193	198	203	208	212	217	222	227	232	237	242	247	252	257	262	267
60	97	102	107	112	118	123	128	133	138	143	148	153	158	163	168	174	179	184	189	194	199	204	209	215	220	225	230	235	240	245	250	255	261	266	271	276
61	100	106	111	116	122	127	132	137	143	148	153	158	164	169	174	180	185	190	195	201	206	211	217	222	227	232	238	243	248	254	259	264	269	275	280	285
62	104	109	115	120	126	131	136	142	147	153	158	164	169	175	180	186	191	196	202	207	213	218	224	229	235	240	246	251	256	262	267	273	278	284	289	295
63	107	113	118	124	130	135	141	146	152	158	163	169	175	180	186	191	197	203	208	214	220	225	231	237	242	248	254	259	265	270	278	282	287	293	299	304
64	110	116	122	128	134	140	145	151	157	163	169	174	180	186	192	197	204	209	215	221	227	232	238	244	250	256	262	267	273	279	285	291	296	302	308	314
65	114	120	126	132	138	144	150	156	162	168	174	180	186	192	198	204	210	216	222	228	234	240	246	252	258	264	270	276	282	288	294	300	306	312	318	324
66	118	124	130	136	142	148	155	161	167	173	179	186	192	198	204	210	216	223	229	235	241	247	253	260	266	272	278	284	291	297	303	309	315	322	328	334
67	121	127	134	140	146	153	159	166	172	178	185	191	198	204	211	217	223	230	236	242	249	255	261	268	274	280	287	293	299	306	312	319	325	331	338	344
68	125	131	138	144	151	158	164	171	177	184	190	197	203	210	216	223	230	236	243	249	256	262	269	276	282	289	295	302	308	315	322	328	335	341	348	354
69	128	135	142	149	155	162	169	176	182	189	196	203	209	216	223	230	236	243	250	257	263	270	277	284	291	297	304	311	318	324	331	338	345	351	358	365
70	132	139	146	153	160	167	174	181	188	195	202	209	216	222	229	236	243	250	257	264	271	278	285	292	299	306	313	320	327	334	341	348	355	362	369	376
71	136	143	150	157	165	172	179	186	193	200	208	215	222	229	236	243	250	257	265	272	279	286	293	301	308	315	322	329	338	343	351	358	365	372	379	386
72	140	147	154	162	169	177	184	191	199	206	213	221	228	235	242	250	258	265	272	279	287	294	302	309	316	324	331	338	346	353	361	368	375	383	390	397
73	144	151	159	166	174	182	189	197	204	212	219	227	235	242	250	257	265	272	280	288	295	302	310	318	325	333	340	348	355	363	371	378	386	393	401	408
74	148	155	163	171	179	186	194	202	210	218	225	233	241	249	256	264	272	280	287	295	303	311	319	326	334	342	350	358	365	373	381	389	396	404	412	420
75	152	160	168	176	184	192	200	208	216	224	232	240	248	256	264	272	279	287	295	303	311	319	327	335	343	351	359	367	375	383	391	399	407	415	423	431
76	156	164	172	180	189	197	205	213	221	230	238	246	254	263	271	279	287	295	304	312	320	328	336	344	353	361	369	377	385	394	402	410	418	426	435	443

Adapted from *Clinical guidelines on the identification, evaluation, and treatment of overweight and obesity in adults: the evidence report.* Accessed at www.nhlbi.nih.gov/guidelines/obesity/bmi_tbl.pdf.

WELL CARD DYSLIPIDEMIA, HYPERGLYCEMIA, HYPERTENSION

Lipid Goals

Total cholesterol	Less than 200 mg/mL
LDL cholesterol[a]	
Low risk	Less than 160 mg/mL
Intermediate risk	Less than 130 mg/mL
High risk[b]	Less than 100 mg/mL
Very high risk	Less than 70 ng/mL
Triglycerides	Less than 150 mg/dL

[a]Goals differ depending on cardiac disease risk.
[b]Automatically if you have heart disease or diabetes.

Blood Sugar Goals

Fasting plasma glucose (FPG)

Normal fasting glucose[a]	Less than 100 mg/mL
Impaired glucose tolerance (pre-diabetes)	100 to 125 mg/mL
Diabetes	126 mg/mL or higher

[a]fasting = no caloric intake for 8 hours.
DM = any FPG over 125 or any random plasma glucose over 199 with symptoms.
Corresponding numbers for oral glucose tolerance test (OGTT) (2-hour postload glucose):
normal = under 140 mg/mL; impaired glucose tolerance (IGT) = 140 to 199 mg/mL;
diabetes = 200 mg/mL or more.

Blood Pressure Goals

Optimal blood pressure	Less than 120/80 mm Hg
Prehypertension	Systolic 120 to 139 mm Hg or diastolic 80 to 89 mm Hg
Hypertension	140/90 mm Hg or higher

Sources

Lipid goals	NCEP-ATP III
Blood sugar	American Diabetes Association
Blood pressure	The Seventh Report of the Joint National Committee on Prevention, Detection, Evaluation, and Treatment of High Blood Pressure (JNC 7).

ADDITIONAL RESOURCES

http://hin.nhlbi.nih.gov/atpiii/calculator.asp?usertype=prof—10-year
cardiac risk calculator

About cholesterol
http://www.nhlbi.nih.gov/guidelines/cholesterol/atglance.pdf—Great
quick desk reference ATP-III (Cholesterol Guidelines)

About diabetes
http://www.diabetes.org/about-diabetes.jsp
http://care.diabetesjournals.org/content/vol29/suppl_1/

About hypertension
http://www.nhlbi.nih.gov/guidelines/hypertension/index.htm
http://www.nhlbi.nih.gov/guidelines/hypertension/phycard.pdf—Great
reference card

WELL CARD METABOLIC SYNDROME

A cluster of metabolic findings that are seen in patients with central obesity: impaired glucose tolerance, hypertension, and dyslipidemia. The metabolic syndrome is an independent risk factor for cardiac disease. It is very common in schizophrenia, 41% in the CATIE cohort (McEvoy et al., 2005).

To diagnosis the metabolic syndrome you need to:
- Measure waist circumference
- Check blood pressure
- Check labs: fasting glucose and lipids

Diagnostic Criteria[a]

Parameter	Value	Yes	No
Waist circumference	Male >40 in. (102 cm) Female >35 in. (88 cm)		
Fasting glucose	≥110 mg/dL		
Blood pressure	≥130/85		
Fasting triglycerides	≥150 mg/dL		
HDL cholesterol	Male ≤40 mg/dL Female ≤50 mg/dL		

[a]You need 3 of 5.

Based on NCEP-ATP III. Other criteria (e.g., World Health Organization criteria) exist, which have different cutoffs or different parameters.

Clinical Pearls

- Lifestyle changes can dramatically improve the metabolic syndrome *even if there is no weight loss.* Encourage regular exercise and reasonable diet (e.g., no soft drinks, no donuts, normal portion size).
- Patients might need medications to lower their cardiac risk.

ADDITIONAL RESOURCES

http://www.nhlbi.nih.gov/guidelines/cholesterol/index.htm—The Cholesterol Guidelines (NCEP-ATP-III criteria) from the National Institutes of Health, National Heart Lung and Blood Institute.

WELL CARD PHYSICAL HEALTH MONITORING IN SCHIZOPHRENIA

	BL	1	2	3	4	5	6	7	8	9	10	11	12
Past medical history and family history	×												×
Smoking status	×	×	×	×	×	×	×	×	×	×	×	×	×
Weight (BMI)	×	×	×	×	×	×	×			×			×
Waist circumference	×												×
Fasting glucose	×			×									×
Fasting lipid profile	×			×									×
Blood pressure	×			×			×						×
Tardive dyskinesia	×						×						×
Medical screening[a]	×												×

[a] Includes review of medical screening needs (e.g., colonoscopy, eye exam), review of vaccination requirements, review of need for testing for infectious diseases (e.g., HIV, hepatitis C virus, tuberculosis).

Note: The numbers in this table indicate number of months

- Recommendations reflect need for increased metabolic monitoring in the initial period after second-generation antipsychotics are instituted.
- More intensive monitoring can be clinically indicated.
- For further guidance, more specific guidelines need to be consulted.

ADDITIONAL RESOURCES

American Diabetes Association, American Psychiatric Association, American Association of Clinical Endocrinologists, et al. Consensus development conference on antipsychotic drugs and obesity and diabetes. Diabetes Care 2004;27: 596–601.

Goff DC, Cather C, Evins AE, et al. Medical morbidity and mortality in schizophrenia: guidelines for psychiatrists. *J Clin Psychiatry* 2005;66:183–194.

Marder SR, Essock SM, Miller AL, et al. Physical health monitoring of patients with schizophrenia. *Am J Psychiatry* 2004;161:1334–1349.

WELL CARD SMOKING CESSATION—DRUG THERAPIES

The following is an exemplary 8-week smoking cessation treatment protocol:

Week −1 or −2	Start bupropion SR 150 qam for three days, then 150 bid
Week 0	**Quit date**
Week 0 to 4	Start nicotine replacement therapy (NRT) Transdermal patch 21 mg[a] every 24 hours Plus PRN NRT (gum/lozenge/inhaler/spray)[b]
Week 5 and 6	Transdermal patch 14 mg every 24 hours
Week 7 and 8	Transdermal patch 7 mg every 24 hours
Week 8	Stop transdermal patch Consider continuing PRN NRT Stop bupropion SR (no need to taper) or consider continuing

[a]If smoking <10 cigarettes per day, start with 14 mg patch.
[b]High-dose NRT (combination NRT = patch plus gum/lozenge/inhaler/spray) unless smoking <10 cigarettes per day.

Drug Therapies

Bupropion

Use bupropion SR 150 mg: one pill for 3 days, then one bid
Main clinical concern: dose-related seizure risk

Nortriptyline

25 mg/day qd × 3 days, then 50 mg/d × 11 days, then 75 mg/day; plasma level week 4

Varenicline (Chantix)

A new nicotinic receptor partial agonist.
Dosing is 0.5 mg for 3 days, then 0.5 mg twice daily for 4 days, then 1 mg twice daily (after a meal); main side effect seems to be gastrointestinal (nausea and vomiting).
Treat for 12 weeks plus additional 12 weeks if successfully quit (to prevent relapse).

Nicotine replacement therapy

Over the counter: gum or lozenges (if heavy smoker use 4 mg, otherwise use 2-mg strength), skin patch (16-hour or 24-hour). Can use lozenges and gum every hour when starting. Chew gum slowly and hold in cheek (to allow for absorption); no acidic beverages (including coffee) 30 minutes around lozenge use (less absorption); skin patch can irritate skin.

Prescription: vapor inhaler, nasal spray. Both are irritating.

WELL CARD SMOKING CESSATION—STAGES OF CHANGE

Based on Prochaska and DiClemente's Transtheoretical Model of Change, patients go through a cycle when they contemplate a behavioral change (like smoking cessation). Five easily identifiable phases provide a framework for tailored interventions. (Some have added a stage prior to the precontemplation phase, "anticontemplation phase" for those who get aggressive if changing is mentioned.)

Precontemplation phase

Patient: "Smoking is not a problem." Patient is in denial, ignorance is bliss.

Intervention: Educate, express concern, and recommend quitting.

Contemplation phase

Patient: "Smoking may be a problem." Patient on the fence, ambivalent, unsure if possible.

Intervention: Have patient list positive and negative things about smoking. Work on barriers.

Preparation phase

Patient: "I want to quit within the next month. Can you help me plan?" Some experimentation with small changes, e.g., smoking less.

Intervention: Set quit date, select strategy (e.g., NRT, bupropion), and muster social support.

Action phase

Patient: "I quit smoking."

Intervention: Contact and support; problem solving around triggers.

Maintenance phase (relapse prevention)

Patient: "I used to smoke."

Intervention: Reinforce benefits of choice made.

ADDITIONAL RESOURCES

Miller WR, Rollnick S, Conforti K. *Motivational Interviewing. Preparing people for change.* 2nd ed. New York: Guilford Press; 2002.—The standard book on the widely used technique of motivational interviewing.

Zimmerman GL, Olsen CG, Bosworth MF. A "stages of change" approach to helping patients change behavior. *Am Fam Physician* 2000;61:1409–1416.—Concise summary of Prochaska and DiClemente's Stages of Change model (aka Transtheoretical Model of Change).

Suggested Readings & Citations

Addington D, Addington J, Patten S, et al. Double-blind, placebo-controlled comparison of the efficacy of sertraline as treatment for a major depressive episode in patients with remitted schizophrenia. *J Clin Psychopharmacol.* 2002;22:20–25.

Adler LA, Rotrosen J, Edson R, et al. Vitamin E treatment for tardive dyskinesia. *Arch Gen Psychiatry.* 1999;56:836–841.

Agid O, Kapur S, Arenovich T, et al. Delayed-onset hypothesis of antipsychotic action: A hypothesis tested and rejected. *Arch Gen Psychiatry.* 2003;60:1228–1235.

Aleman A, Agrawal N, Morgan KD, et al. Insight in psychosis and neuropsychological function: Meta-analysis. *Br J Psychiatry.* 2006; 189:204–212.

Allison DB, Mentore JL, Heo M, et al. Antipsychotic-induced weight gain: A comprehensive research synthesis. *Am J Psychiatry.* 1999; 156:1686–1696.

American Diabetes Association, American Psychiatric Association, American Association of Clinical Endocrinologists, et al. Consensus development conference on antipsychotic drugs and obesity and diabetes. *Diabetes Care.* 2004;27:596–601.

Andreasen NC, Carpenter WT Jr., Kane JM, et al. Remission in schizophrenia: Proposed criteria and rationale for consensus. *Am J Psychiatry.* 2005;162:441–449.

Andreasson S, Allebeck P, Engstrom A, et al. Cannabis and schizophrenia: A longitudinal study of Swedish conscripts. *Lancet.* 1987; 2:1483–1486.

Azorin J-M, Akiskal H, Akiskal K, et al. Is psychosis in DSM-IV mania due to severity? The relevance of selected demographic and comorbid social-phobic features. *Acta Psychiatr Scand.* 2007; 115:29–34.

Bedwell JS, Donnelly RS. Schizotypal personality disorder or prodromal symptoms of schizophrenia? *Schizophr Res.* 2005;80:263–269.

Bilder RM, Goldman RS, Robinson D, et al. Neuropsychology of first-episode schizophrenia: Initial characterization and clinical correlates. *Am J Psychiatry.* 2000;157:549–559.

Branson BM, Handsfield HH, Lampe MA, et al. Revised recommendations for HIV testing of adults, adolescents, and pregnant women in health-care settings. *MMWR Recomm Rep.* 2006;55(RR14):1–17.

Buckley PF, Stahl SM. Pharmacological treatment of negative symptoms of schizophrenia: Therapeutic opportunity or cul-de-sac? *Acta Psychiatr Scand.* 2007;115:93–100.

Carpenter WT Jr. Evidence-based treatment for first-episode schizophrenia [editorial]? *Am J Psychiatry.* 2001;158:1771–1773.

Carpenter WT Jr., Hanlon TE, Heinrichs DW, et al. Continuous versus targeted medication in schizophrenic outpatients: Outcome results. *Am J Psychiatry.* 1990;147:1138–1148.

Carpenter WT Jr., Buchanan RW, Kirkpatrick B, et al. Diazepam treatment of early signs of exacerbation in schizophrenia. *Am J Psychiatry.* 1999;156:299–303.

Chalasani P, Healy D, Morriss R. Presentation and frequency of catatonia in new admissions to two acute psychiatric admission units in India and Wales. *Psychol Med.* 2005;35:1667–1675.

Cooke MA, Peters ER, Kuipers E, et al. Disease, deficit or denial? Models of poor insight in psychosis. *Acta Psychiatr Scand.* 2005;112:4–17.

Correll CU, Leucht S, Kane JM. Lower risk for tardive dyskinesia associated with second-generation antipsychotics: A systematic review of 1-year studies. *Am J Psychiatry.* 2004;161:414–425.

Cournos F, Guido JR, Coomaraswamy S, et al. Sexual activity and risk of HIV infection among patients with schizophrenia. *Am J Psychiatry.* 1994;151:228–232.

Craig D, Mirakhur A, Hart DJ, et al. A cross-sectional study of neuropsychiatric symptoms in 435 patients with Alzheimer's disease. *Am J Geriatr Psychiatry.* 2005;13:460–468.

Crumlish N, Whitty P, Kamali M, et al. Early insight predicts depression and attempted suicide after 4 years in first-episode schizophrenia and schizophreniform disorder. *Acta Psychiatr Scand.* 2005;112:449–455.

Csernansky JG, Mahmoud R, Brenner R, et al. A comparison of risperidone and haloperidol for the prevention of relapse in patients with schizophrenia. *N Engl J Med.* 2002;346:16–22.

David AS. Insight and psychosis. *Br J Psychiatry.* 1990;156:798–808.

Davis JM, Chen N, Glick ID. A meta-analysis of the efficacy of second-generation antipsychotics. *Arch Gen Psychiatry.* 2003;60: 553–564.

Dening TR, Berrios GE. Wilson's disease: Psychiatric symptoms in 195 cases. *Arch Gen Psychiatry.* 1989;46:1126–1134.

de Vries PJ, Honer WG, Kemp PM, et al. Dementia as a complication of schizophrenia. *J Neurol Neurosurg Psychiatry.* 2001;70:588–596.

Douglass AB, Hays P, Pazderka F, et al. Florid refractory schizophrenias that turn out to be treatable variants of HLA-associated narcolepsy. *J Nerv Ment Dis.* 1991;179:12–17.

Emsley R, Rabinowitz T, Medori R. Time course for antipsychotic treatment response in first-episode schizophrenia. *Am J Psychiatry.* 2006;163:743–745.

Essock SM, Covell NH, Davis SM, et al. Effectiveness of switching antipsychotic medications. *Am J Psychiatry.* 2006;163:2090–2095.

Evins AE, Cather C, Deckersbach T, et al. A double-blind placebo-controlled trial of bupropion sustained-release for smoking cessation in schizophrenia. *J Clin Psychopharmacol.* 2005;25:218–225.

Farde L, Wiesel FA, Halldin C, et al. Central D_2-dopamine receptor occupancy in schizophrenic patients treated with antipsychotic drugs. *Arch Gen Psychiatry.* 1988;45:71–76.

Fraunfelder FW. Twice-yearly exams unnecessary for patients taking quetiapine: *Am J Ophthalmol.* 2004;138:870–871.

Freudenreich O. The ABCs of suicide [letter]. *J Clin Psychiatry.* 2005;66:1194–1195.

Freudenreich O, Goff DC. Antipsychotic combination therapy in schizophrenia: A review of efficacy and risks of current combinations. *Acta Psychiatr Scand.* 2002;106:323–330.

Freudenreich O, Goff DC. Polypharmacy in schizophrenia: A fuzzy concept [letter]. *J Clin Psychiatry.* 2003;64:1132.

Freudenreich O, Goff DC. Antipsychotics. In: Ciraulo DA, Shader RI, Greenblatt DJ, eds. *Drug interactions in psychiatry.* 3rd ed. Philadelphia: Lippincott Williams & Wilkins; 2006:177–241.

Freudenreich O, Deckersbach T, Goff DC. Insight into current symptoms of schizophrenia: Association with frontal cortical function and affect. *Acta Psychiatr Scand.* 2004a;110:14–20.

Freudenreich O, Querques J, Kontos N. Checklist psychiatry's effect on psychiatric education [letter]. *Am J Psychiatry.* 2004b;161:930.

Geddes J, Freemantle N, Harrison P, et al. Atypical antipsychotics in the treatment of schizophrenia: Systematic overview and meta-regression analysis. *BMJ.* 2000;321:1371–1376.

Gervin M, Browne S, Lane A, et al. Spontaneous abnormal involuntary movements in first-episode schizophrenia and schizophreniform disorder: Baseline rate in a group of patients from an Irish catchment area. *Am J Psychiatry.* 1998;155: 1202–1206.

Getz K, Hermann B, Seidenberg M, et al. Negative symptoms in temporal lobe epilepsy. *Am J Psychiatry.* 2002;159:644–651.

Ghaemi SN. Hippocrates and Prozac: The controversy about antidepressants in bipolar disorder. *Primary Psychiatry.* 2006;13:51–58.

Ghaemi SN, Hsu DJ, Soldani F, et al. Antidepressants in bipolar disorder: The case for caution. *Bipolar Disord.* 2003;5:421–433.

Gitlin M, Nuechterlein K, Subotnik KL, et al. Clinical outcome following neuroleptic discontinuation in patients with remitted recent-onset schizophrenia. *Am J Psychiatry.* 2001;158:1835–1842.

Glassman AH, Bigger JT Jr. Antipsychotic drugs: Prolonged QTc interval, torsade de pointes, and sudden death. *Am J Psychiatry.* 2001;158:1774–1782.

Goff DC, Cather C, Evins AE, et al. Medical morbidity and mortality in schizophrenia: Guidelines for psychiatrists. *J Clin Psychiatry.* 2005a;66:183–194.

Goff DC, Sullivan LM, McEvoy JP, et al. A comparison of ten-year cardiac risk estimates in schizophrenia patients from the CATIE study and matched controls. *Schizophr Res.* 2005b;80:45–53.

Golomb M. Psychiatric symptoms in metabolic and other genetic disorders: Is our "organic" workup complete? *Harv Rev Psychiatry.* 2002;10:242–248.

Hafner H, Maurer K, Trendler G, et al. Schizophrenia and depression: Challenging the paradigm of two separate diseases—a controlled study of schizophrenia, depression and healthy controls. *Schizophr Res.* 2005;77:11–24.

Harris D, Batki SL. Stimulant psychosis: Symptom profile and acute clinical course. *Am J Addict.* 2000;9:28–37.

Harris EC, Barraclough BM. Excess mortality of mental disorder. *Br J Psychiatry.* 1998;173:11–53.

Henderson DC, Cagliero E, Gray C, et al. Clozapine, diabetes mellitus, weight gain, and lipid abnormalities: A five-year naturalistic study. *Am J Psychiatry.* 2000;157:975–981.

Henderson DC, Cagliero E, Copeland PM, et al. Glucose metabolism in patients with schizophrenia treated with atypical antipsychotic agents: A frequently sampled intravenous glucose tolerance test and minimal model analysis. *Arch Gen Psychiatry.* 2005a;62:19–28.

Henderson DC, Copeland PM, Daley TB, et al. A double-blind, placebo-controlled trial of sibutramine for olanzapine-associated weight gain. *Am J Psychiatry.* 2005b;162:954–962.

Heru AM. Family psychiatry: From research to practice. *Am J Psychiatry.* 2006;163:962–968.

Inouye SK, Bogardus ST Jr. Charpentier PA, et al. A multicomponent intervention to prevent delirium in hospitalized older patients. *N Engl J Med.* 1999;340:669–676.

Johnstone EC, Macmillan JF, Crow TJ. The occurrence of organic disease of possible or probably aetiological significance in a population of 268 cases of first episode schizophrenia. *Psychol Med.* 1987;17:371–379.

Jones PB, Barnes TR, Davies L, et al. Randomized controlled trial of the effect on Quality of Life of second- vs. first-generation antipsychotic drugs in schizophrenia: Cost Utility of the Latest Antipsychotic Drugs in Schizophrenia Study (CUt-LASS 1). *Arch Gen Psychiatry.* 2006;63:1079–1087.

Kane J, Honigfeld G, Singer J, et al. Clozapine for the treatment-resistant schizophrenic: A double-blind comparison with chlorpromazine. *Arch Gen Psychiatry.* 1988;45:789–796.

Kanter J. Engaging significant others: The Tom Sawyer approach to case management. *Psychiatr Serv.* 1996;47:799–801.

Kapur S, Seeman P. Does fast dissociation from the dopamine D(2) receptor explain the action of atypical antipsychotics? A new hypothesis. *Am J Psychiatry.* 2001;158:360–369.

Kapur S, Arenovich T, Agid O, et al. Evidence for onset of antipsychotic effects within the first 24 hours of treatment. *Am J Psychiatry.* 2005;162:939–946.

Katzman GL, Dagher AP, Patronas NJ. Incidental findings on brain magnetic resonance imaging from 1000 asymptomatic volunteers. *JAMA.* 1999;282:36–39.

Kimhy D, Yale S, Goetz RR, et al. The factorial structure of the Schedule for the Deficit Syndrome in schizophrenia. *Schizophr Bull.* 2006; 32:274–278.

Kirkpatrick B, Buchanan RW, Ross DE, et al. A separate disease within the syndrome of schizophrenia. *Arch Gen Psychiatry.* 2001;58: 165–171.

Kirkpatrick B, Fenton WS, Carpenter WT Jr. et al. The NIMH-MATRICS consensus statement on negative symptoms. *Schizophr Bull.* 2006;32:214–219.

Kleinberg DL, Davis JM, de Coster R, et al. Prolactin levels and adverse events in patients treated with risperidone. *J Clin Psychopharmacol.* 1999;19:57–61.

Klerman GL. Psychotropic hedonism vs. pharmacological Calvinism. *Hastings Cent Rep.* 1972;2:1–3.

Koreen AR, Siris SG, Chakos M, et al. Depression in first-episode schizophrenia. *Am J Psychiatry.* 1993;150:1643–1648.

Larsen TK, Melle I, Auestad B, et al. Substance abuse in first-episode non-affective psychosis. *Schizophr Res.* 2006:55–62.

Lehman AF, Kreyenbuhl J, Buchanan RW, et al. The Schizophrenia Patient Outcomes Research Team (PORT): Updated treatment recommendations 2003. *Schizophr Bull.* 2004;30:193–217.

Leucht S, Kissling W, McGrath J. Lithium for schizophrenia revisited: A systematic review and meta-analysis of randomized controlled trials. *J Clin Psychiatry.* 2004;65:177–186.

Levinson DF, Umapathy C, Musthaq M. Treatment of schizoaffective disorder and schizophrenia with mood symptoms. *Am J Psychiatry.* 1999;156:1138–1148.

Liberman RP, Kopelowicz A, Ventura J, et al. Operationalized criteria and factors related to recovery from schizophrenia. *Int Rev Psychiatry.* 2002;14:256–272.

Lieberman JA, Perkins D, Belger A, et al. The early stages of schizophrenia: Speculations on pathogenesis, pathophysiology, and therapeutic approaches. *Biol Psychiatry.* 2001;50:884–897.

Lieberman JA, Stroup TS, McEvoy JP, et al. Effectiveness of antipsychotic drugs in patients with chronic schizophrenia. *N Engl J Med.* 2005a;353:1209–1223.

Lieberman JA, Tollefson GD, Charles C, et al. Antipsychotic drug effects on brain morphology in first-episode psychosis. *Arch Gen Psychiatry.* 2005b;62:361–370.

Lublin FD, Reingold SC. Defining the clinical course of multiple sclerosis: Results of an international survey. National Multiple Sclerosis Society (USA) Advisory Committee on Clinical Trials of New Agents in Multiple Sclerosis. *Neurology.* 1996;46:907–911.

Lubman DI, Velakoulis D, McGorry PD, et al. Incidental radiological findings on brain magnetic resonance imaging in first-episode psychosis and chronic schizophrenia. *Acta Psychiatr Scand.* 2002;106: 331–336.

Lukens TW, Wolf SJ, Edlow JA, et al. Clinical policy: Critical issues in the diagnosis and management of the adult psychiatric patient in the emergency department. *Ann Emerg Med.* 2006;47:79–99.

Manchanda R, Norman R, Malla A, et al. EEG abnormalities and two year outcome in first episode psychosis. *Acta Psychiatr Scand.* 2005;111:208–213.

Marder SR, Essock SM, Miller AL, et al. Physical health monitoring of patients with schizophrenia. *Am J Psychiatry.* 2004;161:1334–1349.

Marneros A. Beyond the Kraepelinian dichotomy: Acute and transient psychotic disorders and the necessity for clinical differentiation [editorial]. *Br J Psychiatry.* 2006;189:1–2.

Marshall M, Lewis S, Lockwood A, et al. Association between duration of untreated psychosis and outcome in cohorts of first-episode patients: A systematic review. *Arch Gen Psychiatry.* 2005;62:975–983.

McEvoy JP, Apperson LJ, Appelbaum PS, et al. Insight in schizophrenia: Its relationship to acute psychopathology. *J Nerv Ment Dis.* 1989;177:43–47.

McEvoy JP, Hogarty GE, Steingard S. Optimal dose of neuroleptic in acute schizophrenia: A controlled study of the neuroleptic threshold and higher haloperidol dose. *Arch Gen Psychiatry.* 1991;48: 739–745.

McEvoy JP, Meyer JM, Goff DC, et al. Prevalence of the metabolic syndrome in patients with schizophrenia: Baseline results from the Clinical Antipsychotic Trials of Intervention Effectiveness (CATIE) schizophrenia trial and comparison with national estimates from NHANES III. *Schizophr Res.* 2005;80:19–32.

McEvoy JP, Lieberman JA, Stroup TS, et al. Effectiveness of clozapine versus olanzapine, quetiapine, and risperidone in patients with chronic schizophrenia who did not respond to prior atypical antipsychotic treatment. *Am J Psychiatry.* 2006;163:600–610.

McGlashan TH, Zipursky RB, Perkins D, et al. Randomized, double-blind trial of olanzapine versus placebo in patients prodromally symptomatic for psychosis. *Am J Psychiatry.* 2006;163:790–799.

McGorry PD, McFarlane C, Patton GC, et al. The prevalence of prodromal features of schizophrenia in adolescence: A preliminary survey. *Acta Psychiatr Scand.* 1995;92:241–249.

McKeith IG, Dickson DW, Lowe J, et al. Diagnosis and management of dementia with Lewy bodies: Third report of the DLB consortium. *Neurology.* 2005;65:1863–1872.

Meltzer HY, Alphs L, Green AI, et al. Clozapine treatment for suicidality in schizophrenia: International Suicide Prevention Trial (InterSePT). *Arch Gen Psychiatry.* 2003;60:82–91.

Menza MA, Murray GM, Holmes VF, et al. Decreased extrapyramidal symptoms with intravenous haloperidol. *J Clin Psychiatry.* 1987;48: 278–280.

Minzenberg MJ, Poole JH, Benton C, et al. Association of anticholinergic load with impairment of complex attention and memory in schizophrenia. *Am J Psychiatry.* 2004;161:116–124.

Mitchell PB, Wilhelm K, Parker G, et al. The clinical features of bipolar depression: A comparison with matched major depressive disorder patients. *J Clin Psychiatry.* 2001;62:212–216.

Murphy KC, Jones LA, Owen MJ. High rates of schizophrenia in adults with velo-cardio-facial syndrome. *Arch Gen Psychiatry.* 1999; 56:940–945.

Naidoo U, Goff DC, Klibanski A. Hyperprolactinemia and bone mineral density: The potential impact of antipsychotic agents. *Psychoneuroendocrinology.* 2003;28 Suppl 2:97–108.

Palmer BA, Pankratz VS, Bostwick JM. The lifetime risk of suicide in schizophrenia: A reexamination. *Arch Gen Psychiatry.* 2005;62: 247–253.

Palmer BW, Heaton RK, Paulsen JS, et al. Is it possible to be schizophrenic yet neuropsychologically normal? *Neuropsychology.* 1997;11:437–446.

Peralta V, Cuesta MJ. Diagnostic significance of Schneider's first-rank symptoms in schizophrenia: Comparative study between schizophrenic and non-schizophrenic psychotic disorders. *Br J Psychiatry.* 1999;174:243–248.

Perkins DO. Predictors of noncompliance in patients with schizophrenia. *J Clin Psychiatry.* 2002;63:1121–1128.

Reilly JL, Harris MS, Keshavan MS, et al. Adverse effects of risperidone on spatial working memory in first-episode schizophrenia. *Arch Gen Psychiatry.* 2006;63:1189–1197.

Rigotti NA. Treatment of tobacco use and dependence. *N Engl J Med.* 2002;346:506–512.

Robinson DG, Woerner MG, McMeniman M, et al. Symptomatic and functional recovery from a first episode of schizophrenia or schizoaffective disorder. *Am J Psychiatry.* 2004;161:473–479.

Rosenheck R, Leslie D, Keefe R, et al. Barriers to employment for people with schizophrenia. *Am J Psychiatry.* 2006;163:411–417.

Rummel C, Kissling W, Leucht S. Antidepressants as add-on treatment to antipsychotics for people with schizophrenia and pronounced negative symptoms: A systematic review of randomized trials. *Schizophr Res.* 2005;80:85–97.

Sachdev P. Schizophrenia-like psychosis and epilepsy: The status of the association. *Am J Psychiatry.* 1998;155:325–336.

Schneider LS, Tariot PN, Dagerman KS, et al. Effectiveness of atypical antipsychotic drugs in patients with Alzheimer's disease. *N Engl J Med.* 2006;355:1525–1538.

Seeman MV. Gender differences in the prescribing of antipsychotic drugs. *Am J Psychiatry.* 2004;161:1324–1333.

Spitzer RL, First MB, Williams JB, et al. Now is the time to retire the term "organic mental disorders." *Am J Psychiatry.* 1992;149:240–244.

Spitzer RL, First MB, Kendler KS, et al. The reliability of three definitions of bizarre delusions. *Am J Psychiatry.* 1993;150:880–884.

Stahl SM, Buckley PF. Negative symptoms of schizophrenia: A problem that will not go away. *Acta Psychiatr Scand.* 2007;115:4–11.

Swanson JW, Swartz MS, Van Dorn RA, et al. A national study of violent behavior in persons with schizophrenia. *Arch Gen Psychiatry.* 2006;63:490–499.

Swartz MS, Wagner HR, Swanson JW, et al. Substance use in persons with schizophrenia: Baseline prevalence and correlates from the NIMH CATIE Study. *J Nerv Ment Dis.* 2006;194:164–172.

Taylor MA, Fink M. Catatonia in psychiatric classification: A home of its own. *Am J Psychiatry.* 2003;160:1233–1241.

van Harten PN, van Trier JC, Horwitz EH, et al. Cocaine as a risk factor for neuroleptic-induced dystonia. *J Clin Psychiatry.* 1998;59: 128–130.

VanderZwaag C, McGee M, McEvoy JP, et al. Response of patients with treatment-refractory schizophrenia to clozapine within three serum level ranges. *Am J Psychiatry.* 1996;153:1579–1584.

Verdoux H, van Os J. Psychotic symptoms in non-clinical populations and the continuum of psychosis. *Schizophr Res.* 2002;54:59–65.

Volavka J, Czobor P, Sheitman B, et al. Clozapine, olanzapine, risperidone, and haloperidol in the treatment of patients with chronic schizophrenia and schizoaffective disorder. *Am J Psychiatry.* 2002;159:255–262.

Vollmer-Larsen A, Jacobsen TB, Hemmingsen R, et al. Schizoaffective disorder—the reliability of its clinical diagnostic use. *Acta Psychiatr Scand.* 2006;113:402–407.

Voruganti LP, Awad AG. Is neuroleptic dysphoria a variant of drug-induced extrapyramidal side effects? *Can J Psychiatry.* 2004;49: 285–289.

Webster R, Holroyd S. Prevalence of psychotic symptoms in delirium. *Psychosomatics.* 2000;41:519–522.

World Health Organization Heads of Centres Collaborating in WHO Co-ordinated Studies on Biological Aspects of Mental Illness. Prophylactic use of anticholinergics in patients with long-term neuroleptic treatment: A consensus statement. *Br J Psychiatry.* 1990;156:412.

Yung AR, Pan Yuen H, McGorry PD, et al. Mapping the onset of psychosis: The Comprehensive Assessment of At-Risk Mental States. *Aust N Z J Psychiatry.* 2005;39:964–971.

Index